This book is for those of you who are grieving and for those who don't always know what to say or do.

With these twenty-six gentle truths, you'll feel less alone and more steady in your life after loss, learning to

live forward

without leaving love behind.

With love and presence,

Lynette Relyea

Please receive this book as a companion that will stay with you long after the services end and the noise fades. It's a quiet way of saying,

"I'm here with you.

You're not alone.

I see you.

I care."

You don't have to carry grief by yourself or move faster than your heart allows.

May these pages keep you company as you discover the Quiet Wow—those surprising moments of comfort that gently remind you love never ends.

Appreciation for "It's Not You, It's Grief"

It's Not You, It's Grief doesn't say, "Do this." It says, "Take what you need. Skip what doesn't fit." Even the subtitle assures me this will not be the all-too-familiar treatment of grief. I read gentle, positive, encouraging words penned by one who has clearly experienced profound sorrow—who has survived it, learned from it, and grown through it. I recognize myself on every page and am heartened to discover that, in time, I will accept the invitation to participate in life again. I am reminded to be patient with myself and to heal at my own pace. How can Lynette's language be so practical and, at the same time, soar?

—Rebecca Middleton, retired missionary and widow

As I read *It's Not You, It's Grief,* Lynette Relyea's practical, warmhearted, and intriguing new book, I found myself engaging in reflection after reflection—on recent change and the loss of siblings, cousins, and my generation; on the surge of saints, relatives, friends, and youth who become comforters along the way; and on the truth that every person grieves differently, and each helps in his own way.

This is not a distant or academic treatment of grief, but a personal, conversational companion—acutely aware of loss, regret, faith, frailty, and hope. It allows space for questions while honoring assurance, patience, and the quiet ways grief can change over time.

—Dwight Reagan, minister

I read *It's Not You, It's Grief* all the way through, and what stayed with me was how gentle it feels. The A–Z format makes it easier to take in when your heart is tired. I liked that it doesn't tell you to hurry up and heal or just pray the pain away. It lets grief be human.

I believe this book is especially for people in those early days after loss, when everything feels unreal and heavy. The words feel comforting and honest, supportive without pushing. It doesn't ask you to be brave or strong—it just sits with you. And sometimes that's what you need most. A quiet reminder that what you're feeling is real, that you're not broken, and that you don't have to walk this alone.

—Eleanor Perry Ford, widow

Having read Lynette's previous books and attended her workshops, I knew to expect compassion—but this book still surprised me. *It's Not You, It's Grief* normalizes emotions in such a powerful way. I appreciated how "A for Acceptance" sets the tone—it feels like the first quiet step, with each letter offering guidance from there. The reflections and journaling give direction without pressure, and the reminder that whatever you do is "enough for today" feels like a gift. Ending with "Z for Zest for Life" felt hopeful and encouraging, like a gentle next step forward. The whole book feels validating, comforting, and deeply human.

—Catherine Larson, constant companion through grief

It's Not You, It's Grief meets grief where it actually lives—in the body, in ritual, in practical decisions, and in the long work of healing. As both a minister and a widower, I recognize the wisdom of a book that honors breath as a daily practice, funerals as personal acts of meaning, gratitude as a sustaining discipline, and uncertainty as "the space where new truths begin to take root." This book offers no formulas—only thoughtful companionship for those learning to live with loss.

—Bill Ehlig, minister and widower

A cold, rainy morning. A loaf of bread in the oven. My fourth cup of coffee, a blanket, and Lynette Relyea's manuscript beside me. That's how I read this book. It felt less like reading and more like being accompanied. These pages meet you in the long after—when the services are over and real life resumes—and offer something rare: steady presence.

—Bella Dion, Managing Partner, Sterling White Funeral Home and Cemetery

I read *It's Not You, It's Grief* from beginning to end because I wanted to learn how to better support others—and I'm so glad I did. It feels supportive and instructive in the best way—gentle, heartfelt, and empowering all at once. Lynette's work brings comfort and hope while honoring the truth that we each have our own work to do.

—Ivory JohnBaptiste, member, Lee College Grief Committee

IT'S NOT YOU,

It's Grief

IT'S NOT YOU, *It's Grief*

Twenty-Six Quiet Truths for Living Forward after Loss

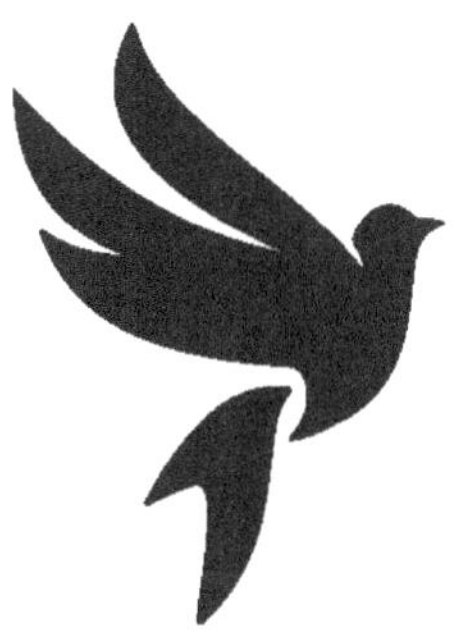

LYNETTE RELYEA

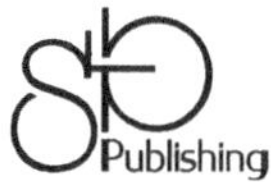

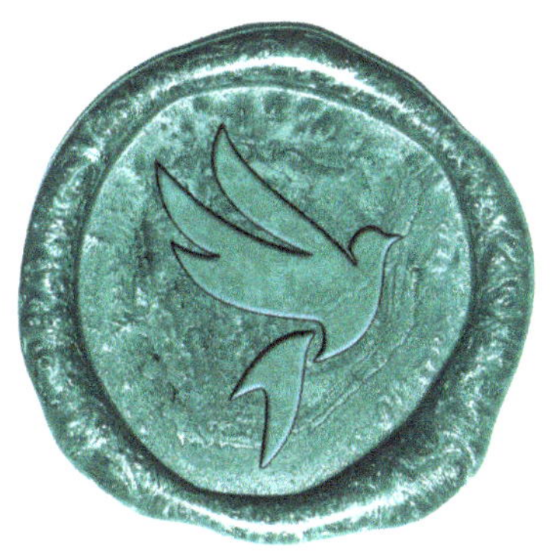

Dedication

Once again, to my Muse, who ignited my heart and whispered, "Let me take you to places you've never been. Your soul knows."

How was I to know what would come after the promise of "till death do us part"—the long after, the grief that would follow love, and the quiet courage it would take to keep living forward without leaving love behind?

The information in this book is offered solely as a support in the reader's personal grief journey after a loss. It is not provided as medical, legal, or psychiatric advice, and neither the author nor the publisher accepts liability related to its use. It is not intended as a substitute for advice from a professional mental health practitioner.

Scott Guerin Publishing
Stewartsville, New Jersey
SG-Publishing.com
guerinscott@gmail.com

Bulk purchases for educational and other purposes can be made by contacting the publisher.

Cover design by Hailee Pavey
Interior design and layout by Hailee Pavey
Pavey Design | paveydesign.com

First Edition: March 2026

ISBN: 979-8-9990391-5-6

Contents

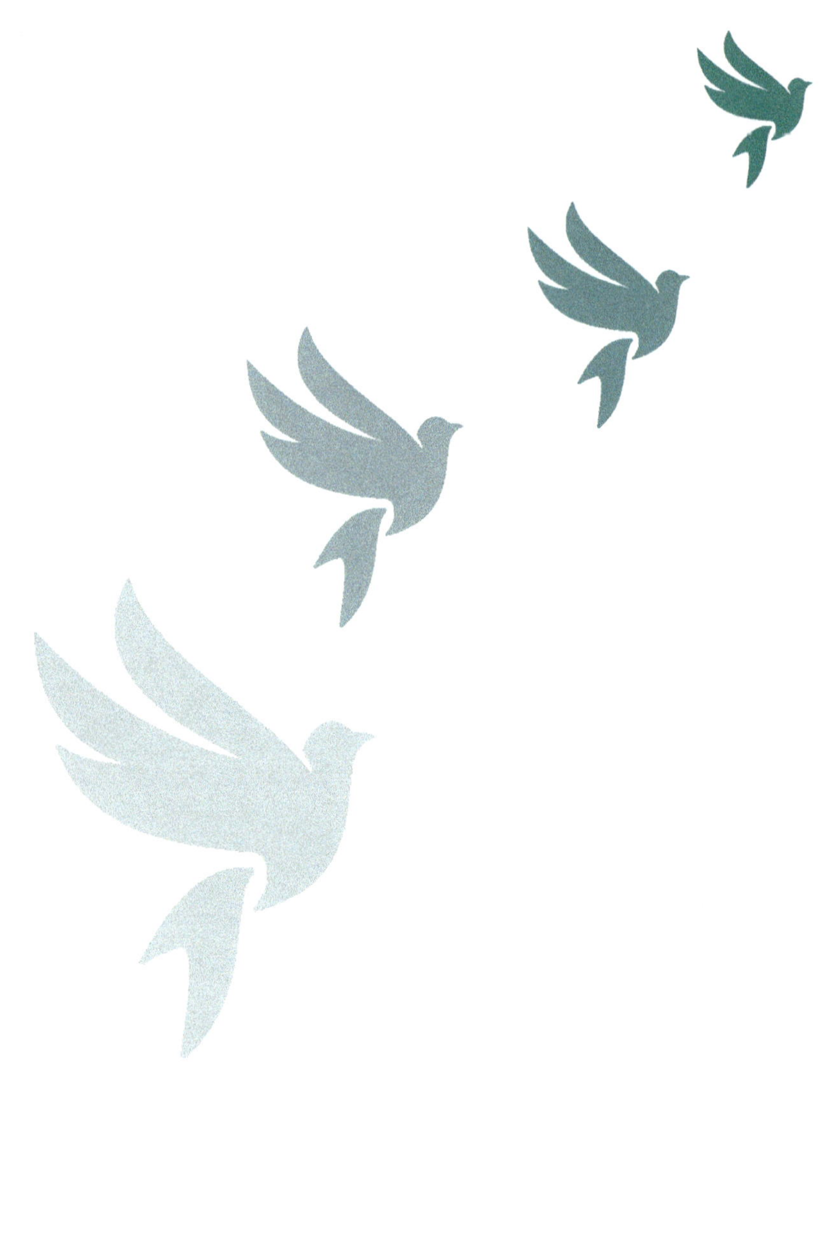

A Blessing for Life after Loss

May this book be a small lantern for the one who has wondered, *Why am I not doing better?*—for the one who has tried so hard and still feels undone.

May it be a gentle witness to what you carry—the love, the missing, the sudden waves, the quiet ache that returns when the world has moved on.

May it softly untie shame from sorrow, so you can breathe again without apologizing for your grief.

May it remind your grieving heart of this truth: this isn't weakness—this is love, continuing.

And when everything feels unsteady, when the days ask more than you have to give, may these twenty-six quiet truths become a steady place to stand.

You are not alone. You are not behind.
You are being held—even here.

Author's Note

This book will not ask you to be strong or move on; it will sit with you in what has changed, help you stay and breathe, and offer you a gentle way to begin again without leaving love behind.

If you are holding this book, you are probably carrying a heavy weight. Please know this: You are not alone.

Grief is brutal. It is a vise crushing your heart.

It is an interrupter, bulldozing the playing field and leaving potholes where there was once solid ground.

It is confusing. It is not wanting to leave where you are and not wanting to go anyplace else.

It is exhausting, unpredictable, overwhelming, all-consuming. Grief affects you physically, intellectually, emotionally, and spiritually.

Your brain is saying, *Do this,* and your heart is saying, *Do that.* But neither one feels fully right.

There is plenty of advice about what to do when a Loved One passes, but where is the helpful guidance for how to live the remainder of your life—the long after—without your Loved One?

You know about power of attorney, preplanning, medical directives, insurance, wills, names on accounts, and numbers on financial documents.

But grief steps in with surprises.

What do you do when your internal GPS is flashing, "Rerouting! Rerouting! Rerouting!"? When the clouds of the long, dark night of the soul cover your north star?

One man told me bluntly, "Grief sucks."

Some days you have only enough energy for the bare minimum—and the bare minimum keeps shrinking. *Maybe tomorrow, if I get around to it,* you think. Getting out of bed is a chore. Eating feels overrated. Sleep is elusive. The only things that you have in abundance are tears and loneliness.

Meanwhile, the world keeps handing you things to deal with—things that need to be done, decisions that need to be made, some practical, some emotional, some spiritual.

And you don't want to deal with any of them—relatives, memories, brain fog, endless questions, overwhelm, holidays, people who mean well but just don't get it, the freezer that goes out and destroys all the food your Loved One prepared for you.

You know there are deadlines. One widow said it this way: "There are so many things I have to do. I feel as if they are all calling me to erase my husband."

You'll know when it's time to open this book. It's not just information. It's a lifeline, a way for me to tell you that you are not alone.

I see you. I care for you. I walk with you as you find your way forward.

You don't have to carry grief alone or move faster than your heart allows.

Slowing down may not be a choice for you, as responsibility, culture, or circumstances require you to keep going, even when your heart is breaking. This book honors that reality, too.

May these pages be a quiet presence as you discover what I call the Quiet Wow, those surprising moments of comfort that remind you that love never ends.

Inside these pages, I highlight a single word or phrase for each letter of the alphabet, with a definition that both names the reality that word encapsulates and offers a compassionate frame for understanding it.

Think of this book as a pocket guide that you can sit with in quiet moments. You don't have to read it all at once or in order. Grief can't be read in a straight line. This book honors that. Let one word speak to you today.

Whether your loss is recent or years behind you, if grief still finds you, you belong here.

In this book, you'll find explanations of common grief experiences such as loneliness, numbness, presence, and guilt. Presence, as I use it here, is the quiet courage to stay—with yourself, with what hurts, with the moment—without needing to fix or explain it. It doesn't make grief disappear; it changes how you carry it.

You'll find a gentle tone—no jargon or heaviness, but no sugarcoating either. Take what you need from these pages. Skip what doesn't fit. Circle back when you are ready.

If you're holding your head in your hands, asking yourself, *What to do? What to do? Where do I even begin?* the first step may surprise you.

Sit in the silence and breathe. Breathe from your heart. Breathe as if your heart itself is breathing. Breathe with your heart until the quiet voice in your heart says, *Okay. You're ready to handle one thing.*

Grief defies labels. It isn't indecisiveness. It isn't laziness. It isn't bemoaning your fate. And it doesn't define you.

This is a time to remember that your grief is uniquely yours. There is no single right way to grieve. This is a time for self-care, a time to be mindful of what and whom you let near your mind, a time to rest, a time for wisdom, a time for discernment.

You are creating Sacred Survival—the practice of living wisely now.

— *Lynette Relyea*

When You Don't Know Where to Turn

You don't need to read this book in order. If your mind feels foggy or your heart feels tender, you may want to begin here.

If you're **feeling overwhelmed or scattered**, you might find steadiness in these entries:

- B—Breathe
- C—Change, Choice, Contemplation
- J—Journey
- U—Uncertainty

If you're **feeling exhausted or depleted,** you may want to rest with the following:

- H—Healing
- P—Patience
- W—Wisdom

If you're **feeling emotionally raw,** these entries may meet you gently:

- E—Emotions
- G—Guilt
- R—Regret
- V—Vulnerability

If you're **feeling alone, unseen, or misunderstood,** you might turn to the following entries:

- N—No Right Way
- O—Others
- S—Support

If you're **facing decisions or responsibilities,** you may want to take refuge in these entries:

- D—Documents
- I—Intention
- M—Money

If your **grief feels long, layered, or ongoing,** you may recognize yourself in these entries:

- K—Keepsakes
- L—Letting Go
- Y—Yearning

If you're **seeking meaning, steadiness, or quiet trust,** you might sit with the following:

- Q—Questions
- T—Trust
- X—Xenia

If you're **sensing a faint return of life,** you may want to begin here:

- Z—Zest for Life

There is no right place to begin—only the place that meets you today.

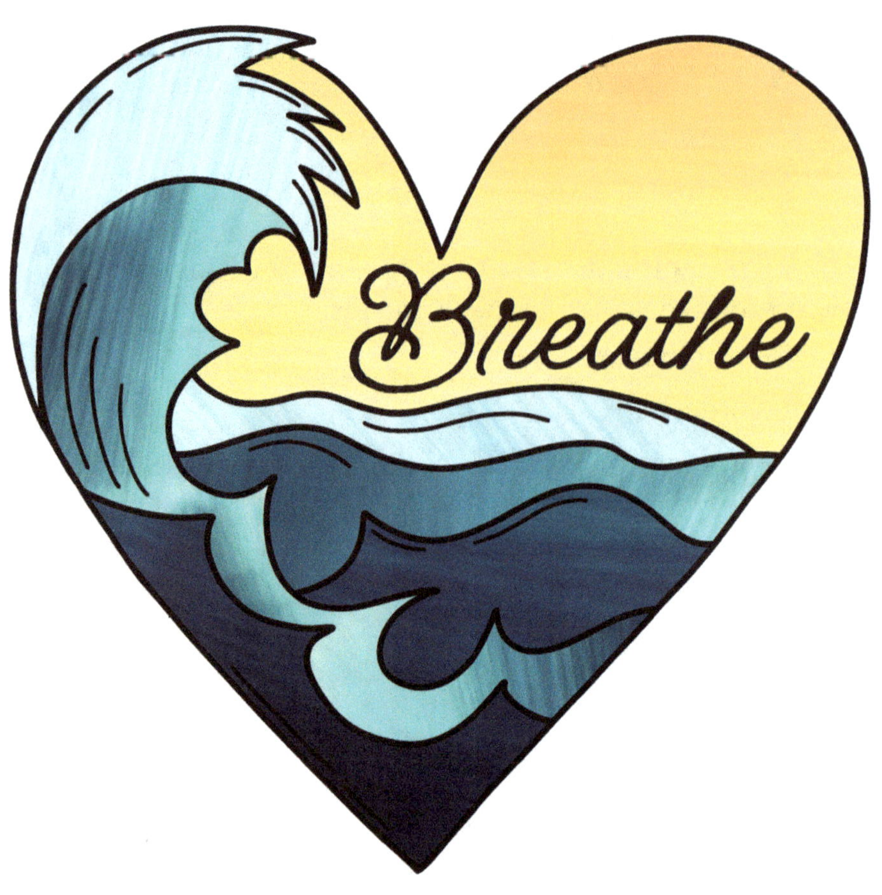

Return to these heart-breath instructions at any point in your journey: when you're feeling overwhelmed, before you begin to journal, or anytime you need to recenter in the midst of daily life.

Before you begin, *breathe from your heart.*

Close your eyes.

Place your hand gently over your physical heart.

Begin to take slow, intentional breaths in through your nose.

Breathe in slowly at your own natural pace.

Feel the rise of your chest, the gentle beat of your heart.

As you exhale through your mouth, more slowly than you inhaled, you are creating a gentle moment of calm amidst the storm.

You don't have to do anything right now—just breathe.

And let your heart speak—not in words, but in a quiet knowing that doesn't need to be explained.

Listen to the silence for what your heart has to tell you.

Stay there as long as you like.

When you're ready, let your pen become a voice for what your heart has whispered.

As you return to the page, bring the calm with you.

Let your next words rise from the quiet place where wisdom lives.

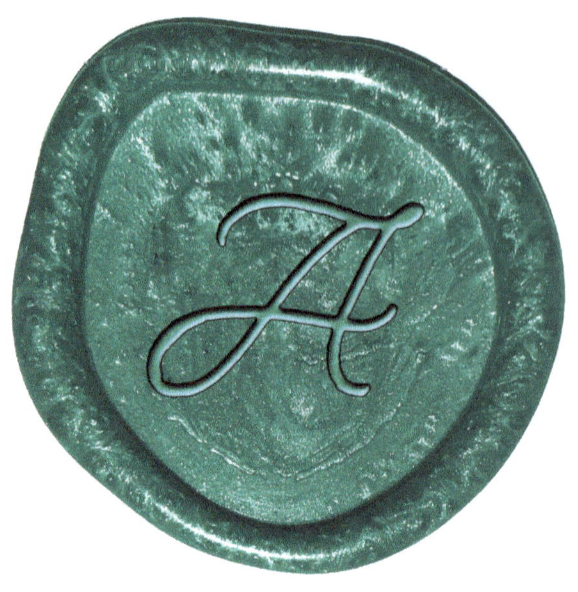

Acceptance

Acceptance does not mean approval.
It simply means that you stop
fighting what is true.

Acceptance is not surrender. It is the quiet moment when the heart stops arguing with truth.

Grief hurts in part because you are clashing with reality. You replay stories about what should have been, what might have been. These stories, though tender and human, can blur the truth. As painful as it is, you must accept that your Loved One is no longer with you in physical form.

Acceptance opens the door to healing and reveals the deeper truths beneath your grief:

> Love endures beyond form.
>
> Peace grows from truth, not from denial.
>
> Healing waits patiently for your willingness to rest in what is, not in what you wish could be.

I release what I cannot change.
I rest in what is true.

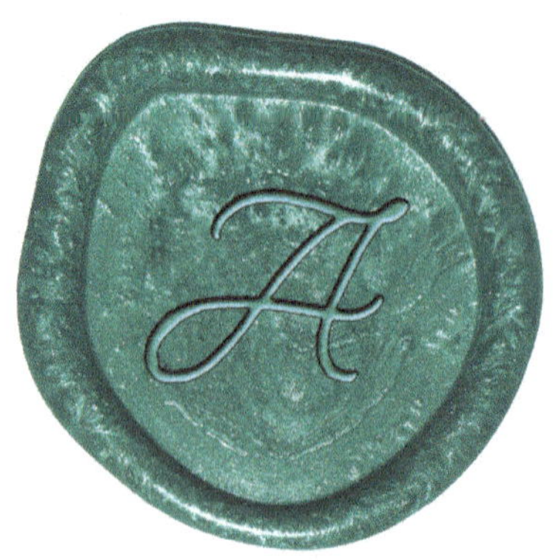

For today, stop arguing with what is true; let your heart rest.

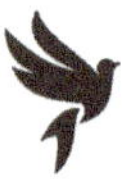

REFLECTION

In what areas am I still fighting a truth that my heart is gently trying to accept?

JOURNAL

What do I notice inside me when I stop resisting what is real and allow myself to rest in what is true today?

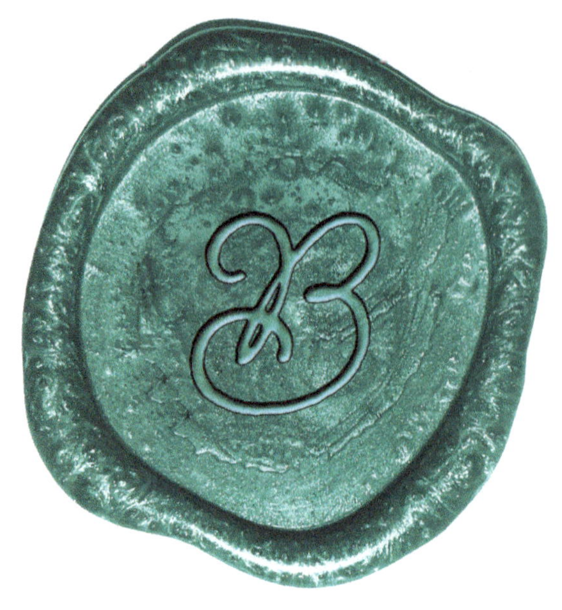

Breathe

When breath returns, life returns—and you remember you are still alive to love.

When you are living in grief, even breathing feels like effort. Your chest tightens. Your breath catches. Your body forgets its rhythm.

Heart breathing is different (see p. 29). It is not a technique. It is a remembering. You invite your heart to lead the way through your grief. You breathe consciously, as if your heart itself is breathing. It is slow, soft, wise, asking nothing of you but presence.

Breath reminds you that calm, comfort, and a flicker of peace can be yours.

And sometimes that is enough for now.

My heart receives the breath of life.
My breath carries me gently through this moment.

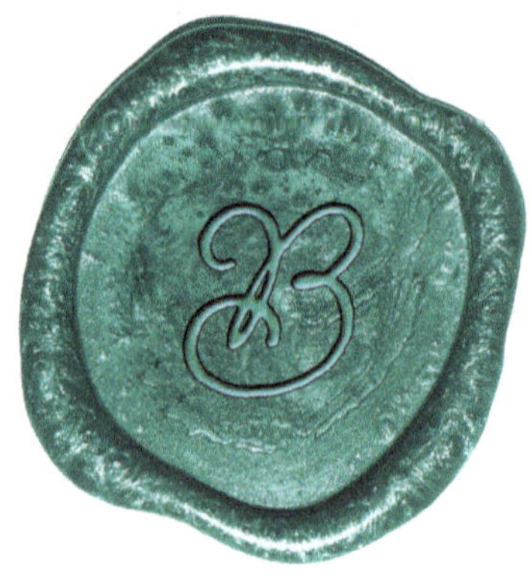

For today, place a hand on your heart and take three slow breaths.

REFLECTION

What do I notice in my body after one slow breath?

JOURNAL

What was a moment when breath spoke kindness to me and helped me feel steady and supported during grief?

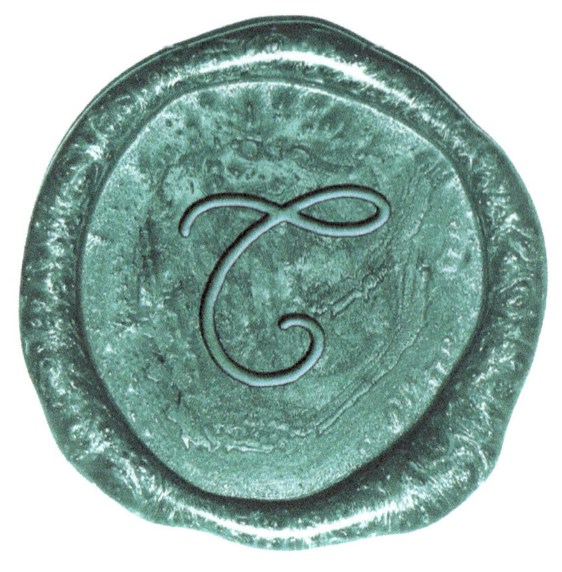

Change, Choice, Contemplation

Change happens to you.
Choice happens through you.
Contemplation happens within you.

Grief begins with the tsunami that changes your world in an instant. Change announces itself on the empty side of the bed, in the silence where laughter once lived, in rearranged calendars, and in the faintest hint of cologne.

Choice is the courage to live in an upside-down world that no longer makes sense. It shows up in the smallest actions: taking a shower on a day when tears come before the water; answering a single text; stepping outside to feel the sky; eating a meal because your Loved One would have wanted that for you; whispering, "I'll try again tomorrow."

Contemplation is the sacred pause between what has changed and what might be possible. It shows up as compassion for yourself, the heart's quiet way of listening for meaning, and truth that no longer needs to be explained. It reveals that the love inside you still wants to move.

I choose with a listening heart.
I let contemplation guide my next step.

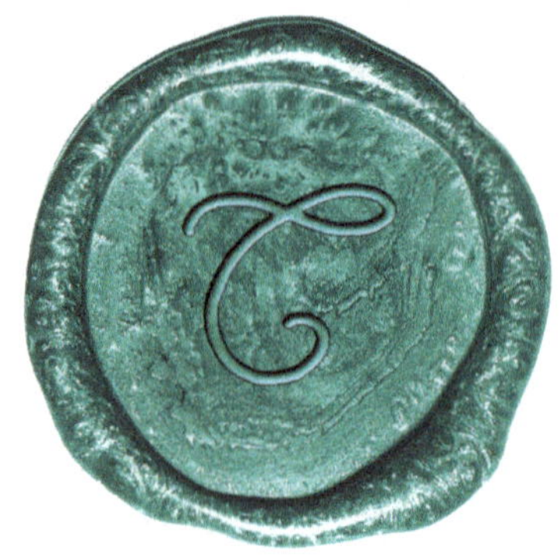

For today, choose one small step; then pause long enough to listen.

REFLECTION

Which recent change feels hardest to acknowledge? What small choice feels possible today?

JOURNAL

What do I notice inside me when I pause long enough to listen for meaning rather than search for answers?

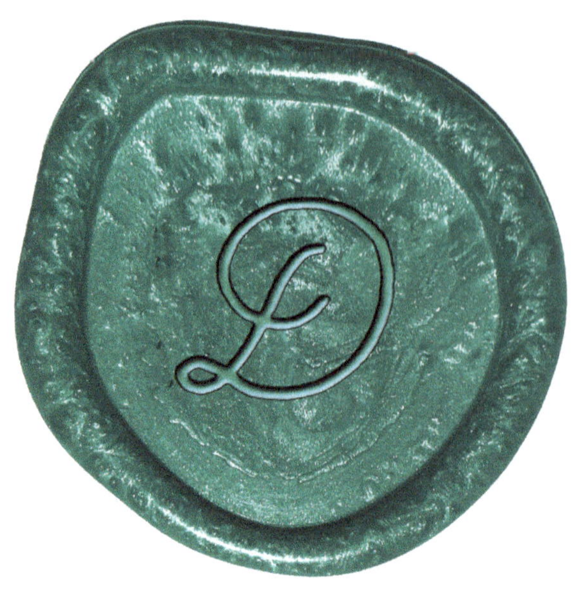

Documents

Documents are the paperwork of loss— the world's way of asking for precision while your heart is learning how to breathe again.

Documents are the endless but necessary papers of loss, and they are exhausting. The world wants information—legal names, dates, account numbers—while you are holding a love that does not fit inside any box on a form.

Each signature feels, as one widow said, as if your Loved One is being erased. It feels like an unwanted acknowledgment of what is now true.

It's not so much the paperwork itself that drains you; rather, it's the emotional labor wrapped in administrative language.

You are not "disorganized." You are grieving, and that makes thinking harder than it used to be.

You are not "behind." You are surviving.

You are not "taking too long." You are honoring the truth that your heart cannot always move at the speed bureaucracy demands.

In this chapter of grief, presence matters more than productivity. Healing cannot be rushed.

Take breaks when you need them. Handle one paper at a time. Breathe between pages.

Let someone sit beside you if that helps. Let someone else handle the task entirely if that's what steadies your heart.

I am doing the best I can.
The world can wait while my heart catches up.

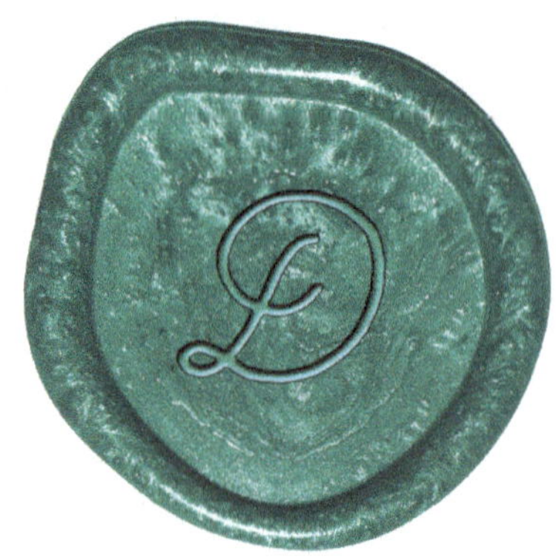

**For today, handle one paper;
then breathe before the next.**

REFLECTION

What do I notice inside me when I face the practical tasks of grief?

JOURNAL

What would it feel like to approach these tasks with compassion and permission for myself instead of pressure?

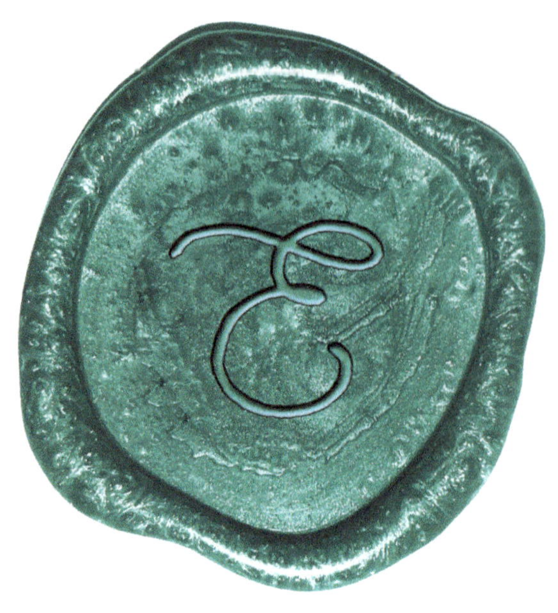

Emotions

Emotions are fragments of love and truth, reminding you of what your mind cannot yet grasp.

Grief confuses the head and overwhelms the heart. Your mind wants to understand, to reason its way through, to find a pattern, to make sense of what has happened. Your heart does not speak the language of logic; it simply wants the ache to stop. Somewhere between the two lies the narrow, sacred space where healing begins—where the head learns to listen and the heart begins to trust again.

What if each emotion—even the sharp, inconvenient ones—is simply trying to tell the truth of your love?

The journey of healing is learning how to let your head and heart listen to each other. The head can say, *This is hard, and it makes sense that it's hard.* The heart can reply, *I am hurting, and I need time.*

Somewhere between them comes compassion—the gentle permission to feel what you feel without apology, without hurry, without judgment. The path between sorrow and peace, though narrow, is still there, and every honest emotion is a step toward it.

I listen to my heart with understanding.
I listen to my head with compassion.

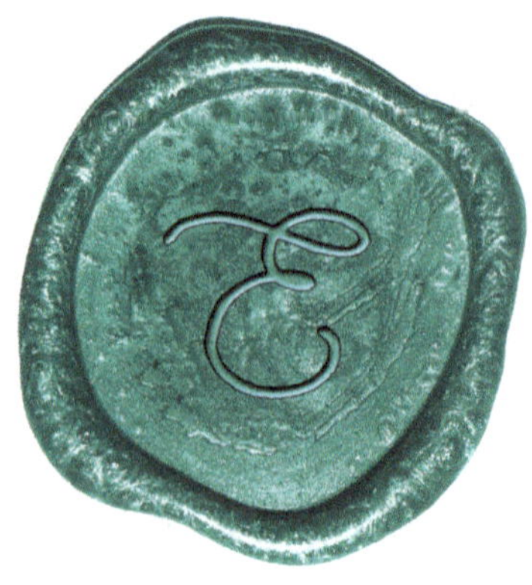

For today, name what you feel without fixing or rushing it.

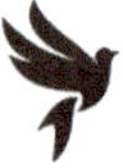

REFLECTION

Which emotion feels closest to the surface right now? What might it be trying to tell me?

JOURNAL

How do my heart and mind speak to each other in this season of grief?

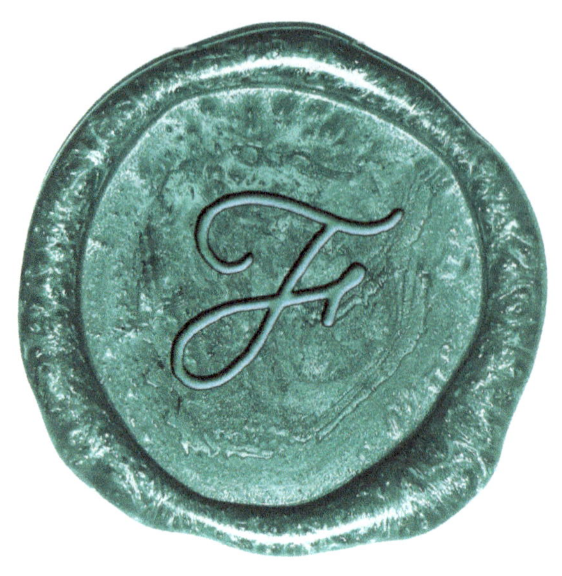

Funeral

A funeral is where love gathers to speak its last earthly language.

A funeral marks what has ended, yet it also reveals what endures. It is both a farewell and a beginning—a ritual of closure and the opening of the long work of carrying love forward.

As a community, we come together not because we know what to say, but because love insists that we show up, even when words fail us. Love gathers us, and in that gathering, every detail feels heavy with meaning—the flowers and traditions, the music that swells, the clothes we choose, the words we can barely speak.

At funerals, presence becomes the truest offering: a hand held, a tear shared, a memory spoken through trembling breath, a nod across the room that says, *I feel this with you.*

If the day feels too much, choose one small way to receive care: a slow breath, or a quiet exit when you need it.

You may think of funerals as a final goodbye, yet for many hearts, they become the first hello of a new kind of relationship—one carried in story, in the quiet presence that remains. A funeral is not an ending. It is a threshold, a sacred moment when the community becomes a witness to both the depth of your loss and the strength of your love.

I honor what was shared.
I carry love forward with grace.

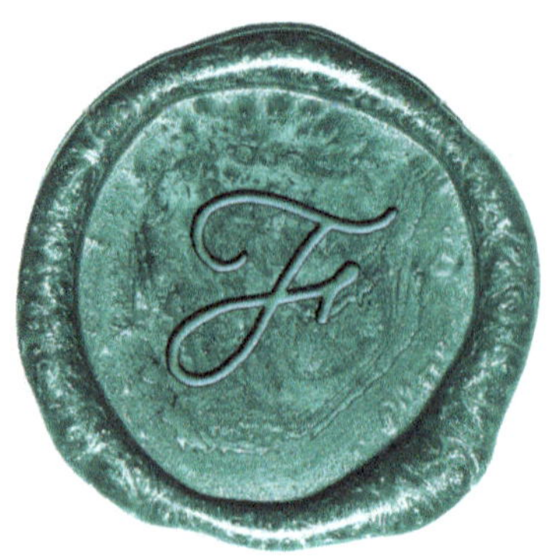

For today, choose one small refuge—a hand, a gentle pause, or a step outside for a breath of fresh air.

REFLECTION

Which moment from my Loved One's funeral or memorial has stayed with me most vividly?

JOURNAL

How did that moment reveal something about love, community, or meaning?

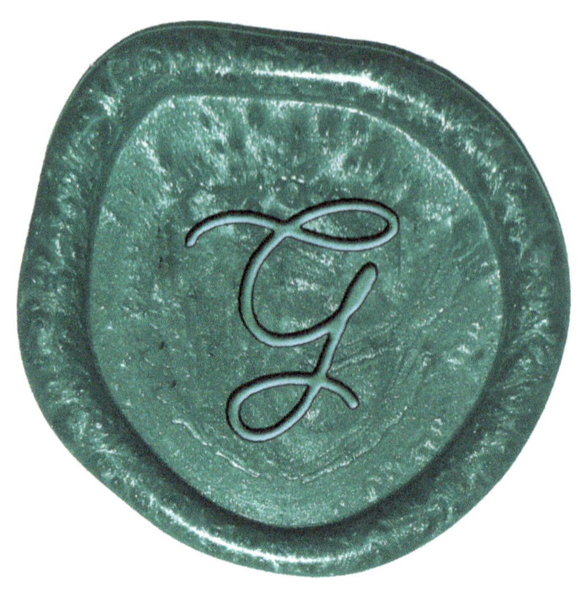

Guilt

Guilt often walks beside grief, whispering what-ifs into an already tender heart.

There are moments when guilt shows up wearing the mask of responsibility. It replays scenes, rewrites endings, and rehearses words you never said. Inside your mind, you hear the haunting refrains of *If only …* and *I should have …*

These thoughts arise because love is trying to make sense of what will never make sense—they are the heart's attempt to control what was never within its power.

Sometimes guilt doesn't come from inside you at all. It drifts in on someone else's words—questions that are meant to bring understanding or help but that quietly land as judgment: "Did the doctors explain what happened?" "Were there any signs you might have missed?" "Have you thought about what you might do differently?" If these words land heavily, that makes sense. Even when asked with care, they can wound a tender heart in grief.

Whether guilt is self-spoken or softly delivered by another, it can drain your energy and cloud the love still surrounding you. Perhaps the work isn't to silence guilt, but to stay present with it—to listen long enough to hear what truth, if any, it carries and to let go of what does not belong.

You begin to heal when you name guilt for what it is: love seeking control in a world that no longer obeys your wishes.

When guilt arises from within, breathe. Remind yourself, *I did the best I could with what I knew at the time.*

When guilt arrives from others, pause. Say inwardly, *That is their need to explain, not my burden to carry.*

I forgive myself for not knowing what I could not know.
I let love speak louder than guilt.

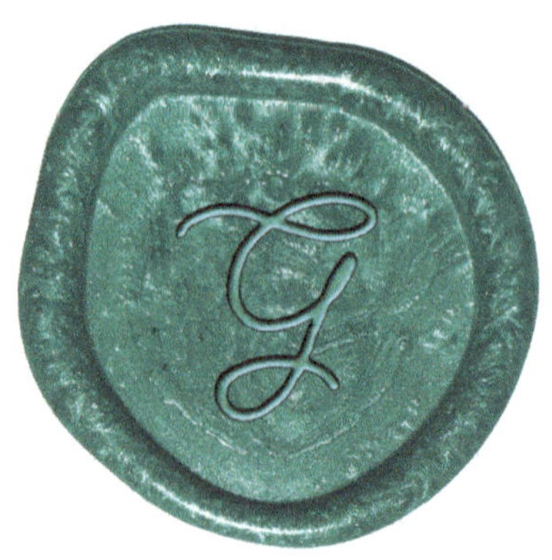

For today, breathe and remind yourself, *I did the best I could.*

REFLECTION

What "if only" thoughts return most often?

JOURNAL

If I spoke to myself with compassion, what truth might soften or release that guilt?

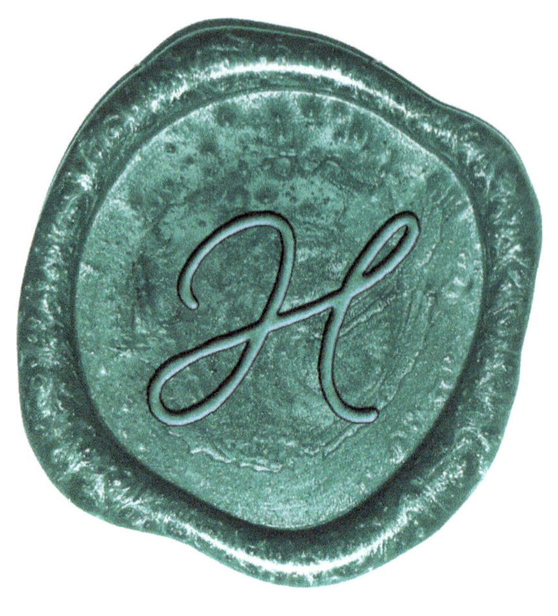

Healing

Healing is not the absence of pain. It is the willingness to be present with what the heart would rather run from.

In grief, healing begins when you stop resisting what hurts and start listening to it.

It begins when you stop asking yourself why and begin asking, *What am I to learn from grief?*

It begins when you notice the small mercies—a breath that brings warmth before tears, a moment of patience you didn't know you had, a sudden laugh that surprises you.

It begins when you realize that healing is less about fixing all that is broken and more about befriending what remains.

It begins when you learn to trust life again in the smallest ways: a cardinal returning to the feeder, a brown rabbit showing up on the patio, a sunset that turns the sky orange, a hand reaching out in kindness, a breath that feels like it might carry you through the next five minutes.

It begins when you no longer let grief define you.

These are not signs that grief has ended. They are proof that love is still alive, that your heart, in its own wise timing, is learning to live alongside the ache.

I am learning to live beside what I've lost.
Peace is finding me, slowly, faithfully.

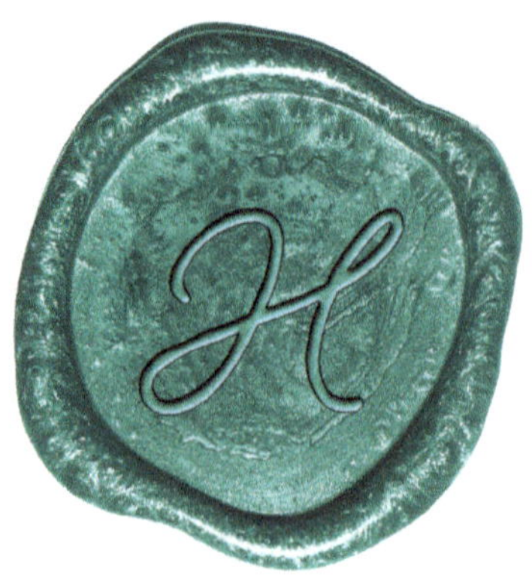

**For today, notice one small mercy—
then let it be enough.**

REFLECTION

Where do I notice tiny signals of healing in myself lately?

JOURNAL

In what ways might healing be inviting me to live alongside my grief, rather than beyond it?

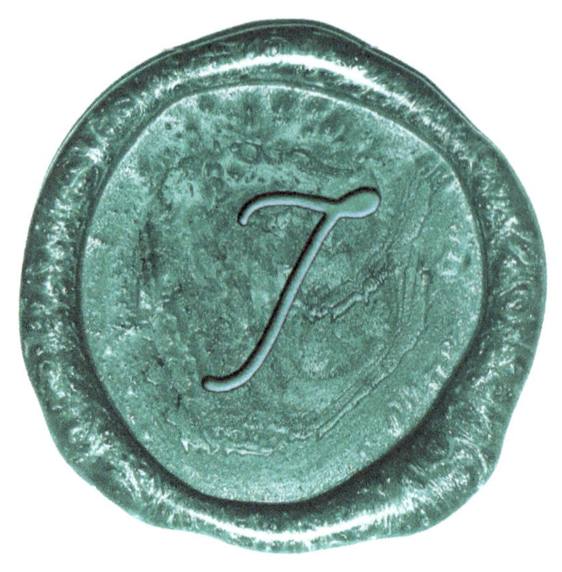

Intention

Intention is love's quiet invitation
to participate in life again
before you feel ready.

Grief shows you what you cannot control. Intention reminds you of what you can control—the way you listen, the way you show up, the way you choose kindness even when your heart feels fragile.

After loss, there comes a day when living begins to whisper again. It starts small—sitting in the sunlight, returning a call, folding the laundry, answering an email, or simply noticing the quiet thought, *I'm tired of being sad.*

These small acts—ones others might overlook—aren't passive endurance. They are acts of courage, even heroic in their own quiet way. Each one is proof that, despite the pain, you keep choosing to show up.

It's not about fixing the past; it's about finding the strength to participate in the present. It's not about erasing grief; it's about living courageously within it. Intention doesn't demand plans or perfection. It asks only for willingness—to keep breathing, to keep noticing, to keep participating in life, one small act at a time.

Intention honors grief by letting love move again—quietly, purposefully—toward life.

I choose to keep showing up.
I move gently toward what still matters.

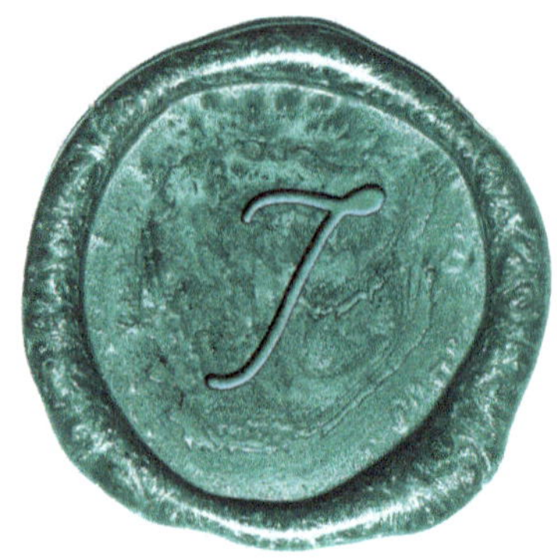

For today, show up for one simple thing that keeps life moving.

REFLECTION

What is one small act of life today that feels doable?

JOURNAL

Was there a moment when I chose to participate in life even while grieving? What made that choice possible?

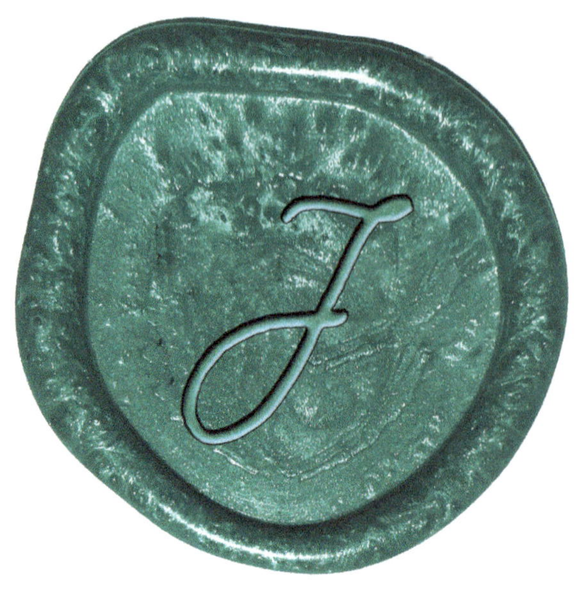

Journey

Grief is not a single moment you endure, but a journey you learn to walk with tender feet.

No one hands you a map for this terrain. There is no compass precise enough to guide a heart that has been broken open.

You stumble through days that blur together. Is this Monday or Tuesday? You start to count on your fingers—your loss measured first in hours, then days, then weeks, months, and years. Has it really been that long?

Some days you walk with purpose; other days you crawl through fog with the headlights on low. Some days you clomp through the swamp. And sometimes you can almost see a faint timberline, a reminder that change is happening, even when you feel stuck.

The path forward is rarely straight. It winds, circles, pauses, and begins again when the heart has strength to move forward. There are no shortcuts, no awards for endurance—only the quiet grace of putting one foot in front of the other. Each step teaches something—patience, grace, the art of breathing from the heart—asking the quiet question, *What am I to learn from this?*

Along the way, grief teaches you to pace yourself. Some steps are heavy with tears. Others carry a fragile hope. You learn that the road itself is the teacher—and your willingness to keep walking is the healing.

The journey of grief is not about leaving love behind. It's about learning how to carry love differently—in story, in memory, in the quiet ways you keep showing up for life.

I walk at the pace my heart allows.
I trust that every step—even the halting ones—is part of healing.

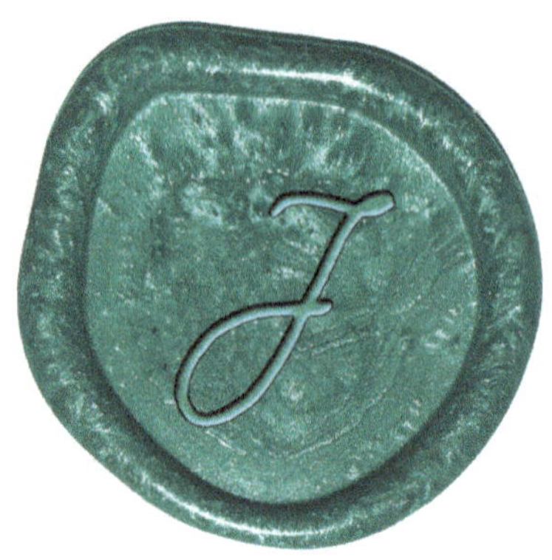

For today, take the next step only—no map required.

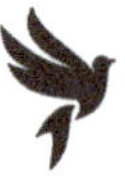

REFLECTION

Where am I on my grief journey right now—moving or pausing?

JOURNAL

What have I learned about myself from walking grief's path at my heart's pace?

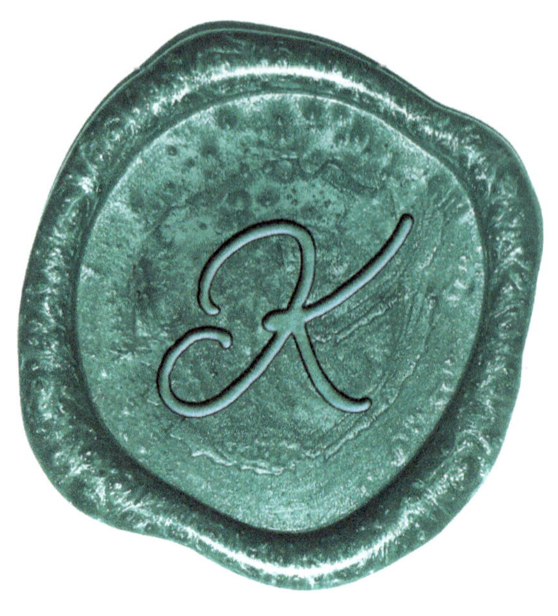

Keepsakes

Keepsakes are the quiet reminders that love can live inside small things.

After loss, even the simplest objects take on a weight you never expected—the watch that is no longer ticking, a sweatshirt from a special vacation, a saved voicemail you cannot bear to delete, a grocery list in your Loved One's familiar handwriting.

These keepsakes become more than belongings. They are traces of a life intertwined with yours. They can comfort and they can overwhelm. They can bring smiles and tears. They can bring joy and aching.

You sort and sift, not because you want to, but because grief asks you to decide what you will carry forward—and what you will bless and let go. This is not the work of decluttering. It is the work of listening to what still matters. You don't have to decide today what to keep forever—only what your heart can hold right now.

A keepsake does not hold the person you loved. It simply holds a moment—a glimpse of who you were together, a whisper that steadies you as you learn to live with what has changed.

I keep what brings peace.
I release what weighs heavy on my heart.

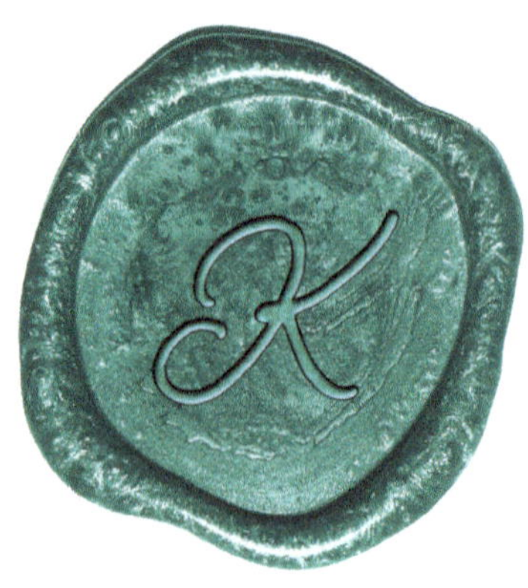

For today, keep only what steadies you; decisions can wait.

REFLECTION

Which items hold emotional weight for me right now? What do they represent?

JOURNAL

What feels right to keep and what might I gently release or bless?

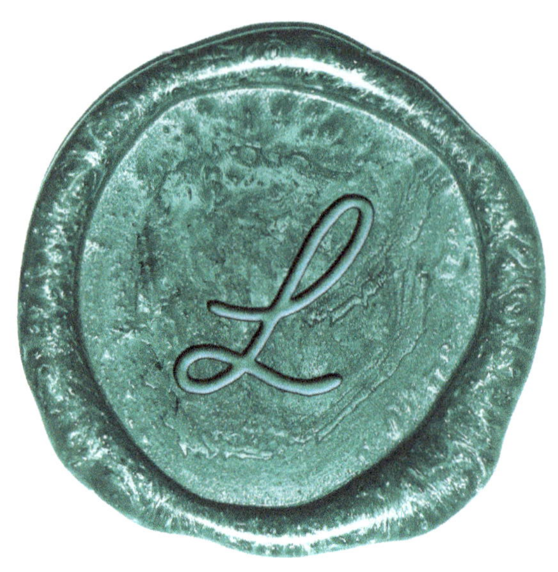

Letting Go

Letting go is not forgetting; it is loosening your grip on what no longer asks to be carried so that your hands and heart can hold what is still alive.

Grief teaches you that holding on and letting go are not opposites. They often show up together.

There are moments when your heart clings tightly to memories, to belongings, to the version of life that made sense before everything changed. And there are moments when something inside you quietly says it's time to release what is keeping you stuck—a ritual, a routine, an expectation, or a responsibility that was never truly yours.

Letting go is not one big moment. It can be as small as loosening your grip for one minute. Letting go is a series of small choices—honest, human, and sometimes reluctant. You let go of timelines that hurry what cannot be hurried. You let go of guilt that was never yours to carry. You let go of expectations—yours and other people's. You let go of roles you assumed out of habit. You let go of the belief that you must grieve in a certain way, or that your healing should look like anyone else's journey.

And when you begin to let go, what's left isn't emptiness. It's space to breathe—space that allows your shoulders to lower and your love to grow when your hands aren't clenched in fear.

I release what is too heavy to hold.
I trust that love remains, even in the letting go.

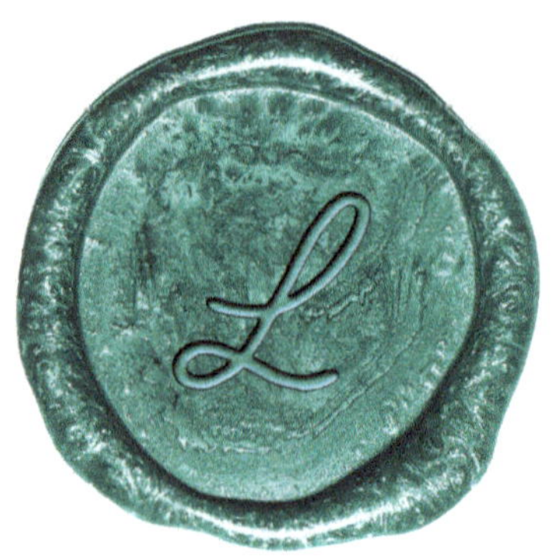

For today, loosen your grip for one breath; that counts as letting go.

REFLECTION

What am I clenching emotionally or mentally that wants softening?

JOURNAL

What would letting go—even just a little—make possible for my heart?

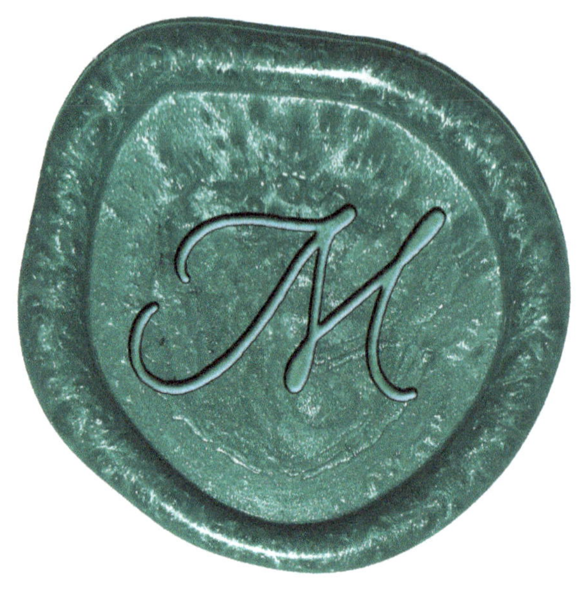

Money

Money becomes heavier after loss—
not just in dollars, but in what it
now represents.

Money in grief isn't just about paying bills or managing accounts. It can stir up questions about security, independence, and self-trust.

It can carry the weight of decisions you never expected to make when the safety of we is gone, decisions about how to keep going when the future feels unfamiliar.

Money after loss often arrives tangled with identity. You may notice old roles shifting—provider, planner, saver, spender, partner. You may question whether you can trust yourself to decide wisely. You may wonder whether asking for help means you have failed. These thoughts are not signs of weakness. They are the mind's attempt to reorient itself after the ground has moved.

Money can also affect relationships. Family members may offer advice you didn't ask for. Support can feel loaded with expectation. You may feel pressure to appear "fine," while inside you are simply trying to understand what this new reality requires of you.

If money feels overwhelming, that makes sense. Grief doesn't just change your heart; it changes how you relate to survival itself.

The gentle truth is this: money does not measure your worth, your intelligence, or your strength. You are allowed to move slowly. You are allowed to postpone decisions that feel too heavy. You are allowed to learn as you go. Needing support—emotional, practical, or professional—is not failure. It is adaptation.

I am doing the best I can. I am allowed to learn as I go. Money does not measure my worth.

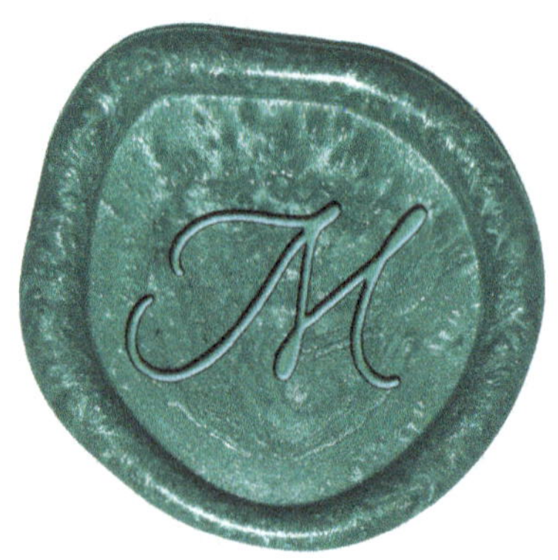

For today, choose one small act that supports your sense of safety—and then let that be enough.

REFLECTION

When I think about money right now, what beliefs about myself come to the surface—capable, uncertain, afraid, steady, something else?

JOURNAL

What story am I telling myself about who I am now in relation to money? Which parts of the story feel kind? Which parts feel harsh?

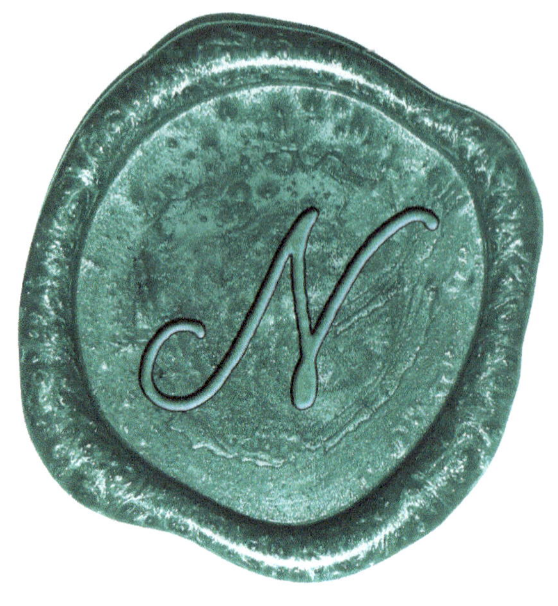

No Right Way

There is no single path through grief; there is only the path your heart has the strength to walk today.

Grief doesn't move in straight lines, even when others expect it to. It doesn't organize itself into neat stages that unfold politely. It certainly does not obey the expectations of people who have never carried your particular loss.

Some days you may feel steady; other days you may fall apart over something small—a song, a scent, a supermarket aisle. You may laugh sooner than you expected or feel nothing long after you thought you "should" feel everything. You may cling to rituals or refuse them. You may talk constantly or say nothing at all.

The way your grief shows up is the way it shows up. There is no wrong way to miss someone. There is no wrong way to love them still. Your grief is as unique as the relationship you lost.

Yet we live in a world that wants grief to look familiar—predictable, orderly, polite. People may offer timelines or opinions about how you're grieving or not grieving, often without realizing that their words can feel like pressure to a heart already carrying so much.

Their expectations cannot define you or measure your love. Your grief does not need permission. The heart that loved is the heart that gets to decide how to mourn. The pace at which you move, the things you keep, the ways you cry, the times you cannot cry—all of it is part of the honest terrain of being human in loss. And if your life doesn't allow you to slow down, you're still not failing.

Your heart knows what it needs. Trust that.

I honor the way my heart is grieving.
I give myself permission to heal in my own time.

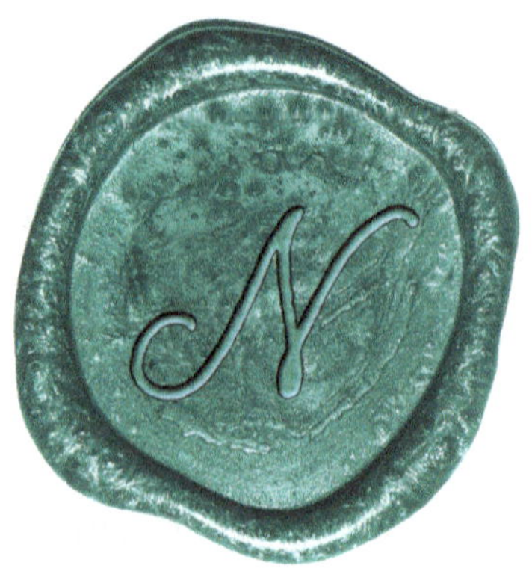

For today, let your grief be yours—exactly as it is.

REFLECTION

Where have I judged myself for grieving "incorrectly"?

JOURNAL

How might I honor my grief as an expression of love rather than a measure of progress?

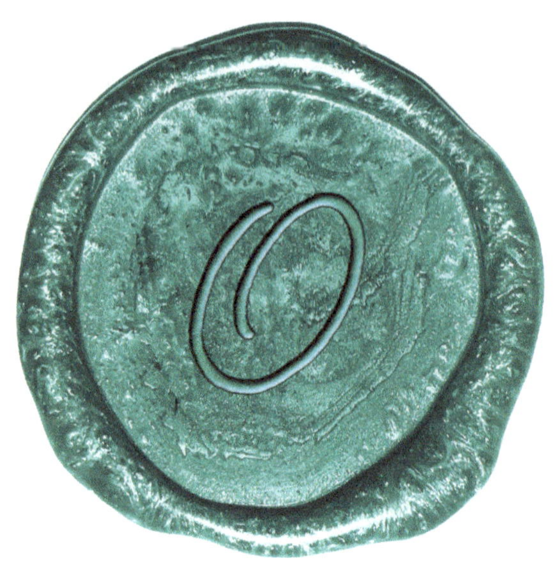

Others

Loss changes your relationships—who shows up, who steps back, and who surprises you altogether.

Grief shows you quickly that not everyone can walk beside you in the same way.

Some people gather close with meals and gentleness.

Some call or text or whisper, "I'm here. I don't know what to say, but I'm here."

Others pull away, not because they don't care, but because your grief stirs something in them that they do not yet know how to face.

Some offer true comfort, while others offer clichés that don't help.

Some need you to be "okay" so that you can make them feel better.

Some offer silence, which can be its own kind of confusing, painful wound.

Here is what grief makes clear: People come with their own fears, histories, and capacities. Not everyone can support you in the way they might want to—or in the way you need. And that is okay.

In all of this, you learn a necessary truth: You can meet others with grace without carrying what is not yours. This means allowing yourself to receive support from those who can offer it and gently stepping back from what feels too heavy. You get to choose who has access to your healing and what feels nourishing to you. You do not have to carry anyone else's expectations while you are grieving.

I welcome those who show up with care.
I release what does not support my healing.

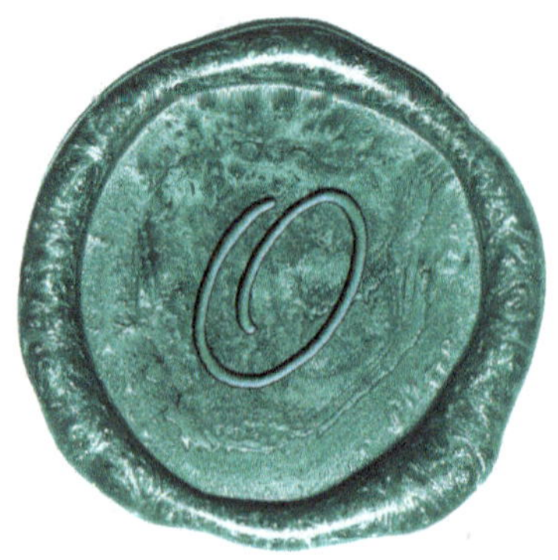

For today, lean toward what feels steady and step back from what drains you.

REFLECTION

Who feels steady and supportive right now?
Who feels heavy or draining?

JOURNAL

How can I receive support from those who show up with care and release what does not help me heal?

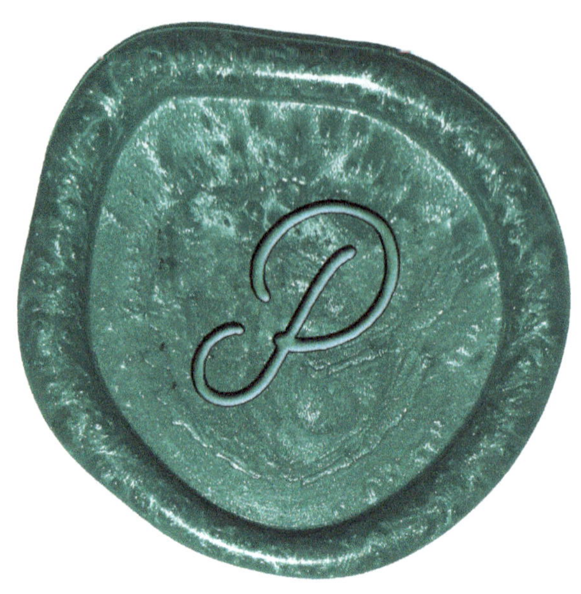

Patience

Patience in grief is not waiting quietly; it is giving your heart the time and space to breathe in a world that has been changed by loss.

Grief asks more of you than you ever expected. Some days move slowly. Some days stretch you beyond what you have to give. Some days don't make sense at all.

You may wonder why you aren't "further along," why a memory still brings tears, or why something small can open the ache you thought had settled. But grief does not follow a calendar or a plan. It follows the tenderness of your own heart, one moment at a time.

Patience is not pushing yourself. It is not pretending you are okay. It is not trying to feel ready before you are. And if rest isn't accessible in your life right now, patience may look like tiny pauses—one breath, one boundary, one softer expectation.

Patience means letting your feelings come and go at their own pace. It means listening when your heart says, *Today I can only take one step.* It means trusting that you are doing the best you can with what your heart can hold.

I give myself time to heal.
I move at the pace my heart allows.

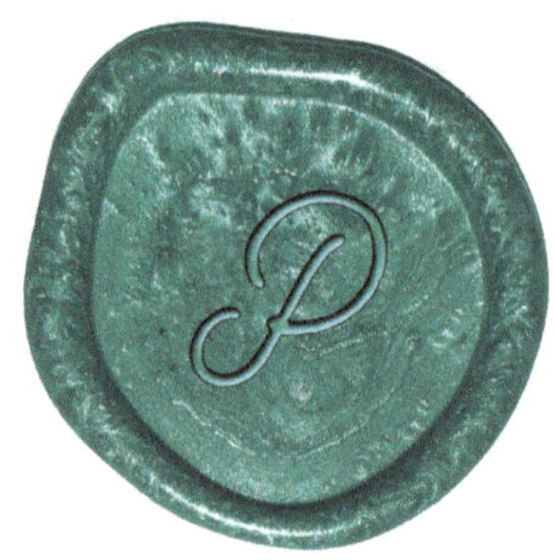

For today, move at the pace your heart allows—nothing faster.

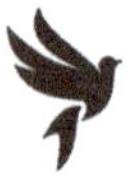

REFLECTION

What would it look like to let my heart set the pace today?

JOURNAL

Where can I offer myself patience instead of pressure?

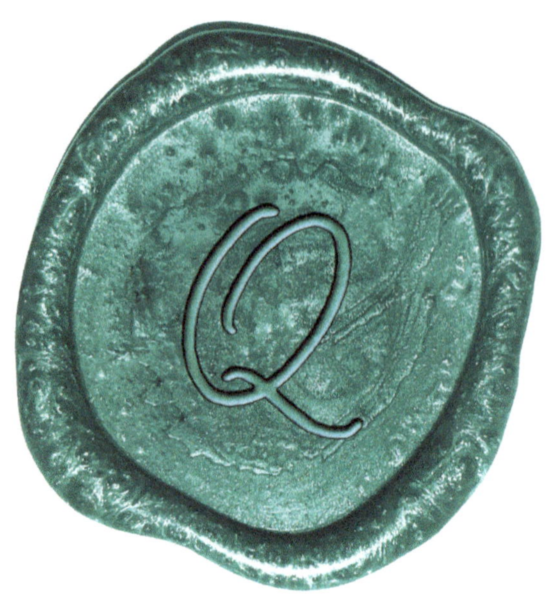

Questions

Grief fills your life with questions—some you can answer, some you cannot, and some that reshape you simply by being asked.

After loss, questions multiply: Why did this happen? Could I have prevented it? What am I supposed to do now? How do I live in a world my Loved One no longer inhabits?

These questions do not arise from confusion. They arise because love is trying to understand what the heart cannot yet bear. Who am I without my Loved One? What still matters? What has changed in me? What do I now know that I did not know before?

Some questions will soften over time. Some will never be answered. Some will reveal wisdom only when the heart is strong enough to hear it.

Grief does not require you to answer every question. It asks you to be patient with them—to let them unfold, to let them teach, to let them be companions rather than burdens. You are allowed not to know, to live forward by continuing to show up for your life, even without full understanding. In time, questions may become guideposts, reminding you of your resilience, your courage, your capacity to hold both sorrow and meaning.

I allow my questions to unfold in their own time.
I trust that clarity will come when I am ready.

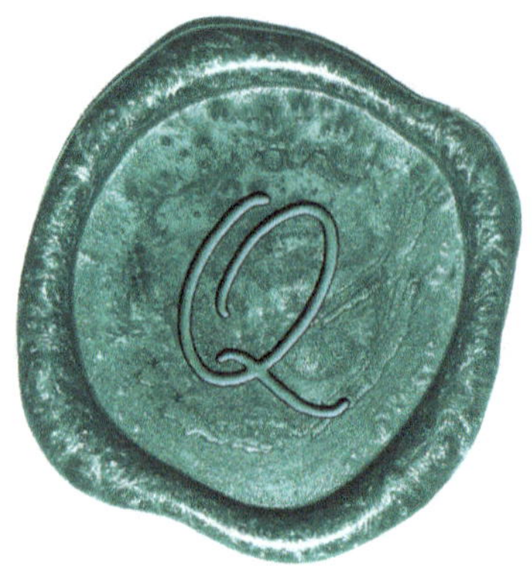

For today, hold one question gently. You don't have to answer it.

REFLECTION

What question is living in me right now? Is it one that cannot be answered but still needs to be heard?

JOURNAL

I will write that question down and allow it to unfold without forcing an explanation.

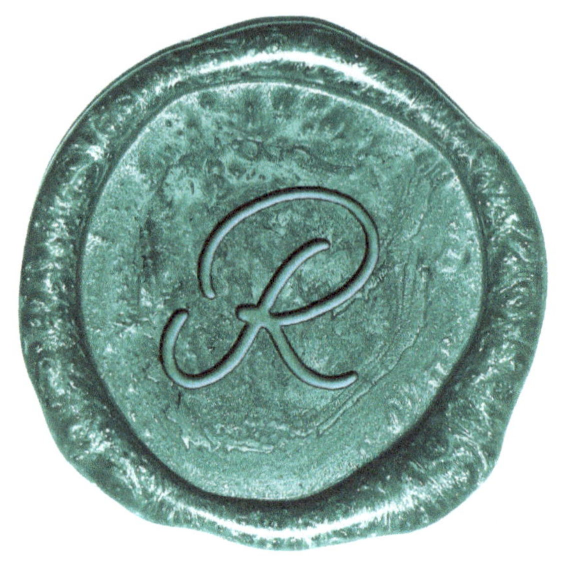

Regret

Regret is the ache of love looking backward, trying to rewrite a story that ended too soon.

In the quiet hours, grief whispers, *I should have known. I should have said more. I should have done something differently. I should have been there sooner. I should have seen what I couldn't possibly have seen. I should have ... I should have ...*

Regret imagines alternate endings because the heart cannot bear the finality of the one it was given. But regret is not truth. It is grief's way of searching for control in a world that no longer feels predictable or safe.

When viewed with compassion, regret reveals something deeper: You loved greatly. You wished you could have protected what was precious. You care more than your heart has words for.

If you listen carefully, you hear, *What am I afraid of? What am I blaming myself for that was never mine to carry? What does this regret reveal about the depth of my love?* If your love story was complicated, regret may arise from both tenderness and incompletion—and you deserve compassion for all of it.

Regret is grief-born tenderness still trying to make meaning from what the mind cannot comprehend. Your task is not to argue with regret, banish it, or silence it. Your task is to meet it with presence: *I hear you. I know you are trying to protect me, but I release what was never mine to control.*

I release the belief that regret is proof of failure.
I allow love to be stronger than regret.

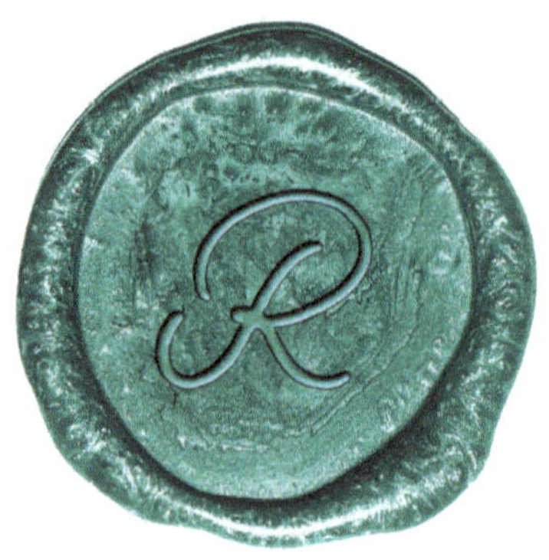

For today, meet regret with compassion, and release what you couldn't control.

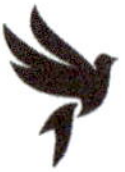

REFLECTION

Which regret visits me most often?

JOURNAL

What would it mean to forgive myself for being human in this moment?

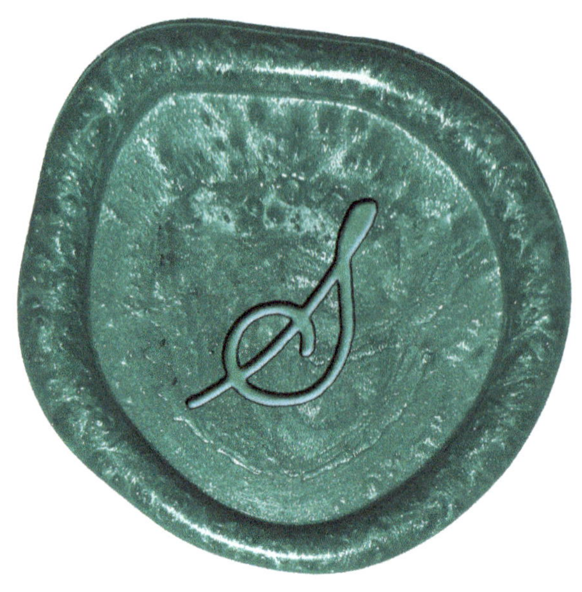

Support

Support in grief is not about fixing what hurts. It is about being held while you learn how to live with what has changed.

After loss, your need for support becomes both deeper and more complex. You may long for comfort yet feel overwhelmed by attention. You may crave connection yet retreat into solitude. You may want to ask for help yet feel unsure what help even means right now.

Support is not one-size-fits-all. It is a living, shifting relationship between your heart's capacity and the presence of others.

True support can look like someone sitting beside you without needing to fill the silence; a friend who listens without offering solutions; a voice that says, "Take your time—I'm not going anywhere"; an act of kindness that requires nothing in return.

And here is an often-overlooked truth: Receiving support is its own form of courage. To let someone witness your vulnerability is to trust that your heart deserves softness. To ask for help is to acknowledge that grief is too heavy to carry alone. To say, "This is what I need," is to honor your healing with clarity and truth.

But not all support feels supportive. Some people show up with advice instead of presence. Some offer words that miss the mark because they fear their own discomfort more than your pain. Discernment becomes essential. You are allowed to say yes to what feels nourishing and no to what feels heavy. You are allowed to choose the companions who will walk with you.

I welcome support that honors my heart.
I release what does not help me heal.

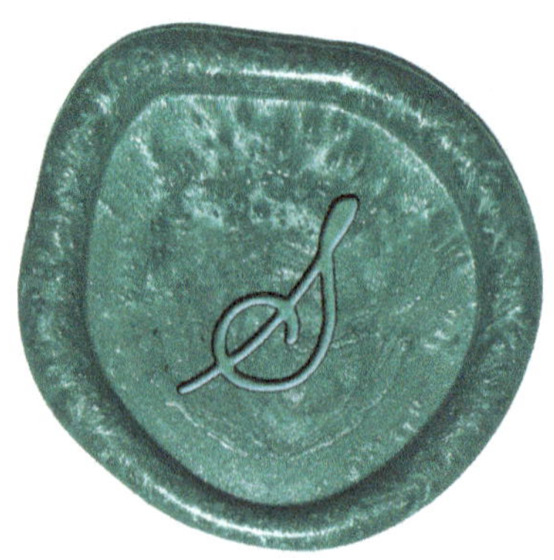

For today, allow one person to be present with you—no explaining, no performing.

REFLECTION

What kind of support does my heart most need today?

JOURNAL

What makes it difficult—or healing—for me to ask for or receive support?

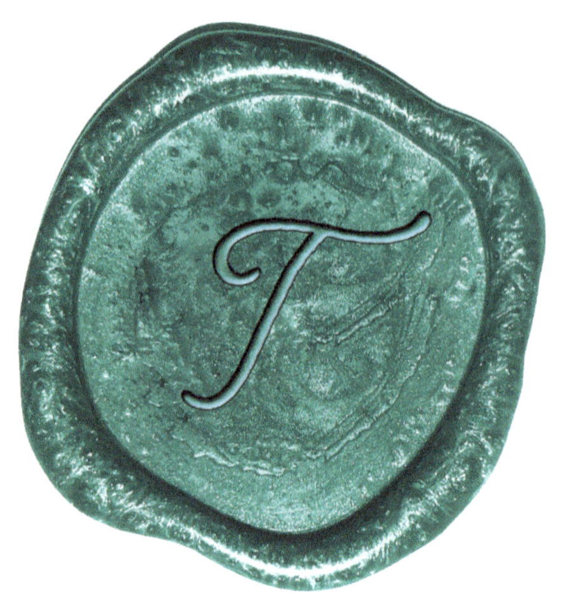

Trust

Trust after loss is not certainty restored.
It is the quiet courage to
take life's hand again even while
your heart is still trembling.

When someone you love dies, trust shatters in many ways: trust in your ability to protect what you cherish; trust you once had in yourself, your intuition, your decisions, your judgment, even your joy; trust in a world that allows such heartache. What once felt solid now feels fragile. What once felt predictable feels uncertain.

Trust doesn't break in one place—it breaks in layers. And it returns the same way. The signs that trust is being rebuilt are so quiet that it's possible to miss them. Trust begins in the smallest gestures: getting out of bed without forcing yourself, listening to your inner wisdom instead of external pressure, taking a breath that feels spacious instead of tight, allowing a moment of softness toward yourself that doesn't need to be earned, making a decision that feels grounded not panicked, experiencing a flicker of hope that doesn't frighten you.

Over time, trust shifts from something you have lost to something you practice with yourself. It grows when you honor your quiet instinct that healing is happening, even beneath the ache. It strengthens when you set boundaries. It deepens when you discern that your resilience is not the absence of grief but the presence of strength within it.

Trust is not the closure of grief. It is the reopening of your relationship with life.

I trust my heart to guide me.
I trust life to meet me gently as I heal.

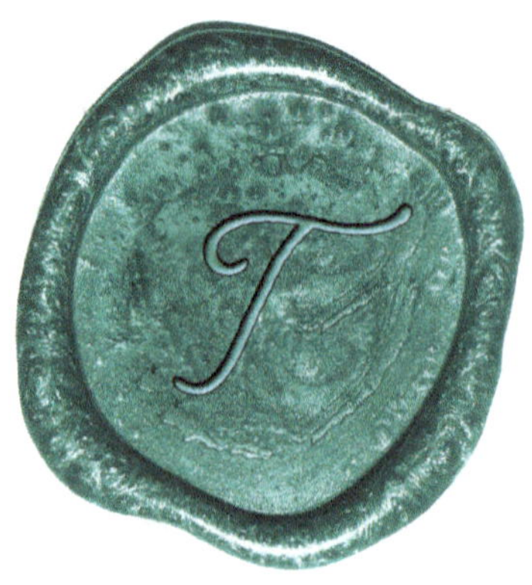

For today, trust returns in small moments. Watch for one.

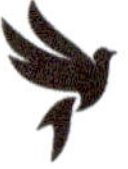

REFLECTION

Where has my trust felt shaken since my loss?

JOURNAL

What small evidence have I seen, however subtle, that my trust is beginning to be rebuilt?

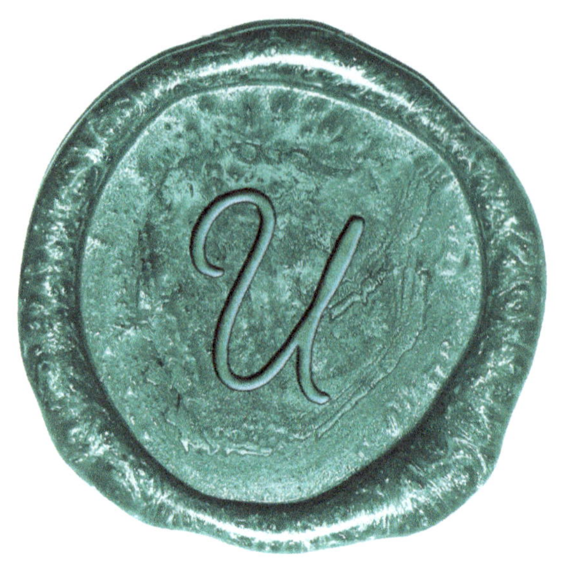

Uncertainty

Uncertainty is the landscape grief paints around you—a terrain where nothing feels familiar and everything asks to be relearned.

After loss, the world becomes a place of unknowns. The routines that once steadied you now feel foreign. The future that once seemed clear dissolves into fog. Even simple choices—what to eat, whom to call, whether to get out of bed—can feel like stepping into a room without a light switch.

Uncertainty is not weakness. It is the honest result of having had your life shaken at its deepest foundation.

The questions come in waves: What am I now? What comes next? How do I live in a world that has lost its shape? Will joy return? Who will I be when it does? These questions are not problems to solve. They are the evidence of a heart trying to reorient itself after losing its north star.

Grief asks you to live without clarity longer than you think you can. But here is the quiet mercy: uncertainty is also the space where new truths begin to take root. In uncertainty, you learn to take one step instead of planning a hundred; to trust the moment rather than the map; to ask what is the best next thing your heart can manage today; to let life reveal itself slowly; to accept that healing is not linear, predictable, or prompt.

Uncertainty is not a void. It is a season of becoming, a sacred in-between in which your old life has ended and your new one is quietly finding its way.

I accept the uncertainty of this season.
I trust that clarity will return in its own time.

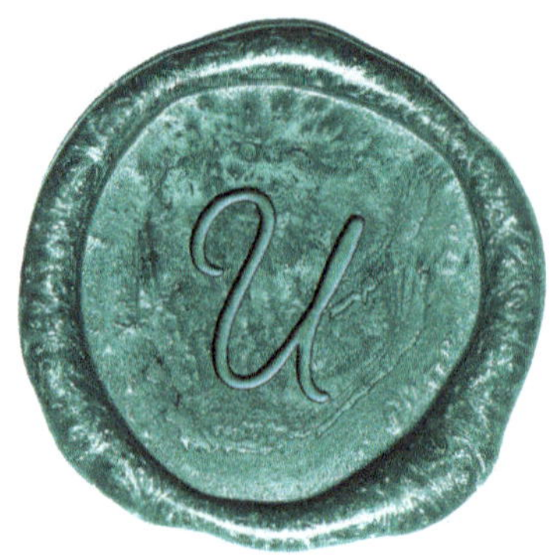

For today, choose the best next step your heart can manage.

REFLECTION

What feels most uncertain for me right now?

JOURNAL

What would it feel like to take just the best next step rather than seeking the whole path?

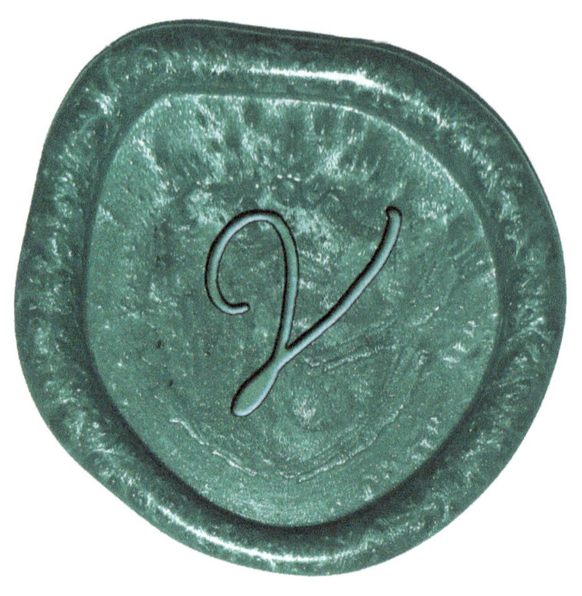

Vulnerability

Vulnerability is not the breaking of strength.

It is the revealing of truth— the soft, unguarded places where love and loss meet.

Grief strips away your defenses. It removes the layers you once relied on to feel steady, safe, composed, and in control. Suddenly, you find yourself crying in the grocery store, staring at the empty side of the bed, forgetting simple tasks, or dissolving at the sound of a familiar song. The openness can feel frightening, as if there is no place left to hide what hurts.

But vulnerability is not exposure; it is honesty.

It is the heart saying, *This is where it hurts. This is where love lived. This is where I am still having a hard time breathing.*

Vulnerability invites a different kind of healing, the kind that comes when you stop pretending to be stronger than you feel. It invites connection: when someone meets your tears with their own; when a friend sits beside you without asking you to be "better"; when you finally say, "I'm not okay," and someone replies, "You don't have to be"; when shared sorrow becomes shared humanity.

Vulnerability creates openings where presence—the kind that doesn't fix or rush or explain—can flow in. It softens what has hardened. It makes space for comfort, for truth, for breath.

Vulnerability is a form of courage—the courage to show up as you are in a world that once held you differently. It's a portal to connection, meaning, and the kind of healing that only grows in the soil of honesty.

I allow myself to be seen as I am.
My vulnerability is a doorway to healing.

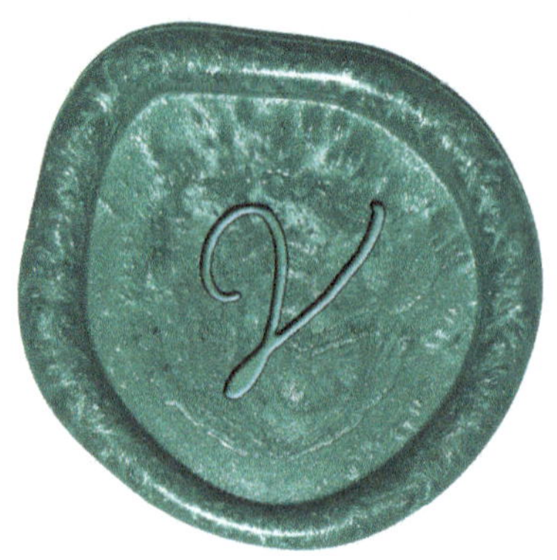

For today, let yourself be real with one safe person.

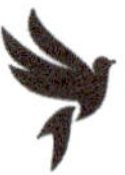

REFLECTION

When have I allowed myself to be seen in my grief? What happened?

JOURNAL

How might vulnerability open a doorway to connection or healing?

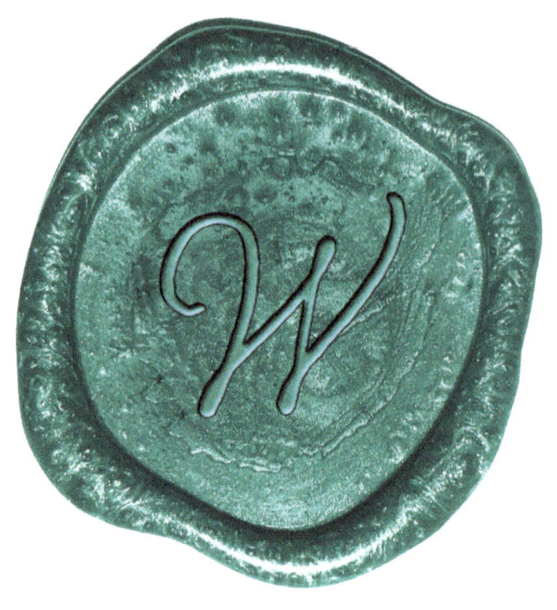

Wisdom

Wisdom is grief's most unexpected gift—the quiet knowing that arises from a heart that has been broken open and still chooses presence.

Wisdom doesn't justify your loss; it simply meets you inside it. You do not seek wisdom in grief. You seek relief, breath, one moment that does not ache. If wisdom feels too far away today, let breath be enough for now.

But over time, as your heart breathes around your loss, something begins to shift. Heartbreak becomes insight. Suffering becomes understanding. Loss becomes a teacher.

Wisdom arrives slowly, like dawn spreading across a dark horizon. It rarely comes as answers. It comes as clarity about what matters and what never truly did. It comes as discernment about who and what can hold your heart and what needs to be let go. It comes as a soul-deep knowing of the difference between noise and truth. It comes as a quiet reverence for time and for the sacredness of ordinary moments. And it comes with an awareness of how you can honor your Loved One—not only with memory, but also with the choices you make as you continue to live.

I welcome the wisdom that is emerging.
I trust the quiet truths grief is revealing.

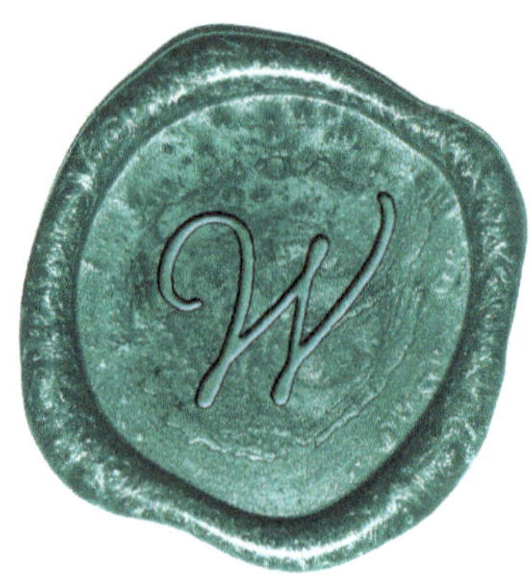

For today, let breath be enough; wisdom can arrive later.

REFLECTION

What has grief taught me—gently or painfully—about myself or about love?

JOURNAL

What was a moment when insight, clarity, or meaning emerged, even in the midst of my sorrow?

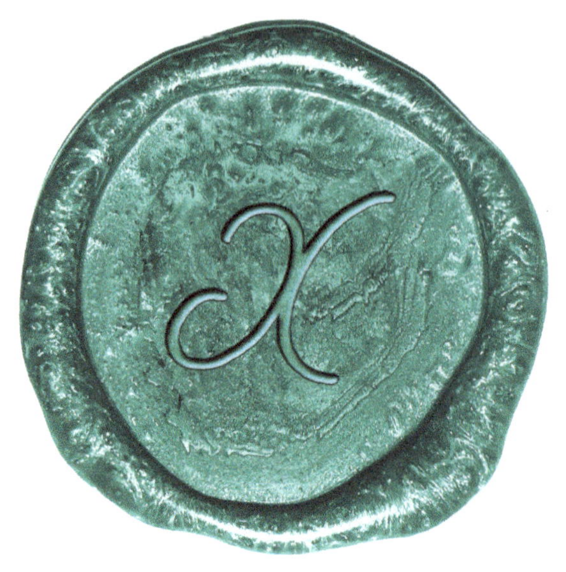

Xenia

Xenia—sacred hospitality—is the ancient practice of offering welcome to the stranger, greeting what arrives with gentleness. In grief, the stranger is often your own heart.

Loss changes you in ways you never anticipated. You look in the mirror and see someone familiar, yet everything inside you feels foreign. Your emotions come in unfamiliar shapes. Your reactions surprise you. Even your voice—the one inside your own head—sounds different.

Xenia, or sacred hospitality, invites you to become a guest in the house of your own soul. You don't have to force yourself back into who you were. Instead, extend hospitality to yourself: Open the door gently instead of demanding that you "go back to normal." Offer yourself a seat at the table of your own compassion. Nourish emotions that arrive hungry and trust that they have something true to reveal. Rest the parts of you that feel weary. Claim warmth for moments that feel cold or abandoned. Declare patience for the heart that is doing its best to survive.

Xenia turns your inner world into a place where the stranger becomes known and understood. It creates a place where healing can sit down and stay awhile.

I offer my heart hospitality.
I welcome what is true in me with gentleness.

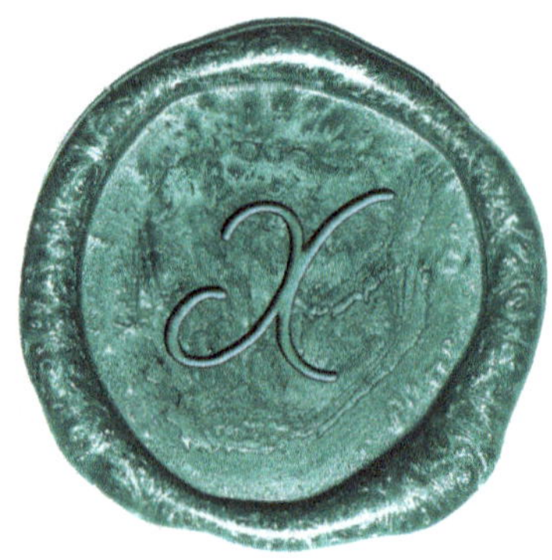

For today, welcome your heart kindly, like a guest who needs warmth.

REFLECTION

How do I respond when my emotions arrive uninvited?

JOURNAL

What would it look like to offer myself hospitality—a soft seat at the table of my own compassion?

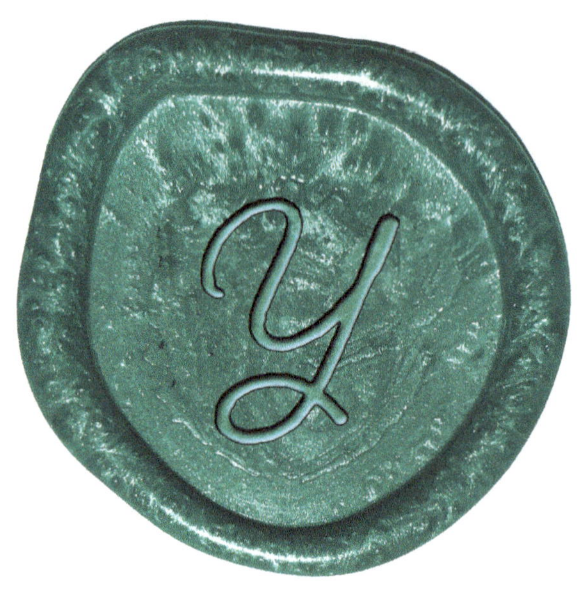

Yearning

Yearning is the echo of love reaching for what it can no longer touch—an ache so strong that it feels etched into the bones.

In grief, yearning arrives without warning. It arises in the quiet moments—in the empty chair; the unmade side of the bed; the routine you still perform out of habit; the instinct to call your Loved One's name; the impossible wish for one more conversation, one more embrace, one more ordinary moment that you now realize was extraordinary.

Yearning is not an indication that you are "stuck." Rather, it can be an affirmation of the truth that you loved deeply—and still do—and that love does not vanish simply because the world has changed. Yearning is love in its rawest form, a natural expression of love reaching across the distance, searching for the one it holds dear.

When yearning arises, place a hand over your heart and breathe. Love is still here.

I honor the yearning of my heart.
It reminds me how deeply I have loved.

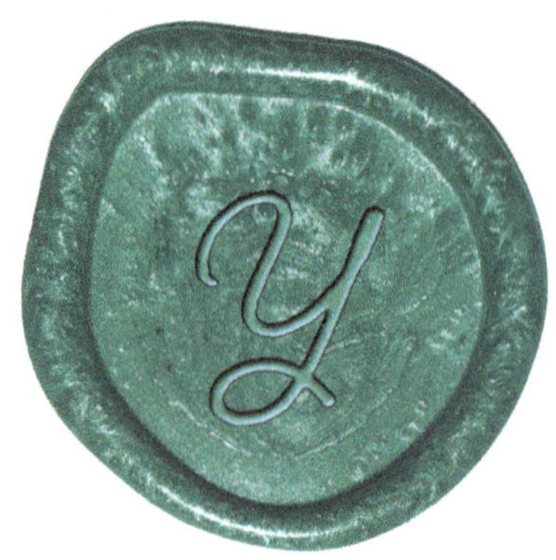

For today, place your hand on your heart and take one slow breath. Love is still here.

REFLECTION

What do I long for most when I think of my Loved One?

JOURNAL

How has yearning shown me the depth and shape of my love?

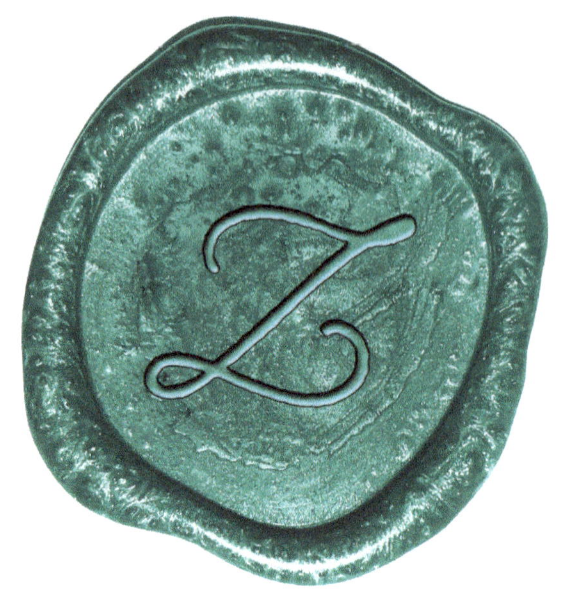

Zest for Life

Zest for life does not return all at once. It returns in faint sparks—small, surprising moments when your heart remembers what it feels like to be fully alive.

In the early seasons of grief, joy feels distant, almost impossible. Your senses seem muted. Your energy is thin. Your capacity for wonder is dimmed by sorrow.

But life has a way of whispering itself back to you. It begins quietly—a laugh that escapes before you can stop it, a sunrise that pulls you toward the window, a meal that tastes good for the first time in months, a song that stirs something other than aching, a moment of curiosity.

Zest for life does not mean forgetting. It means remembering that your heart is capable of more than sorrow, that joy and grief can sit at the same table, and that you can live with one hand holding loss and the other reaching gently toward possibility.

This return to life is not loud or flashy, but rooted, honest, and earned. It is not a leap; it is a series of invitations: Come outside. Be willing to be surprised. Be curious about the future. Try this. Notice that. Stay open. Let life meet you halfway. Hold beauty again. Make room for joy. Let love express itself through the life you continue to live.

I welcome the small sparks of life returning.
My heart is learning to live, fully and tenderly, once more.

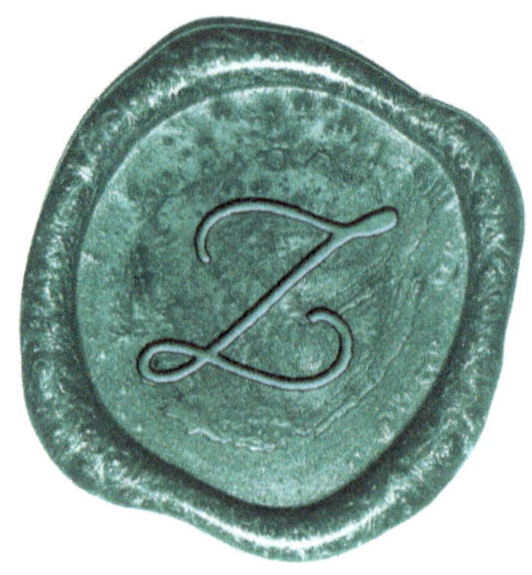

For today, notice one spark of life, however small, and let it stay.

REFLECTION

Where have I noticed even the faintest spark of life returning?

JOURNAL

What small invitation toward life feels possible for me this week?

Acknowledgments

This book was written for the ones living the long after—the ones who wake up to a world that has changed and keep breathing anyway.

First, my deepest gratitude to Bella Dion, who suggested that I write this book. Thank you for seeing what wanted to be said—and for believing it could become a companion for others.

To Susan Davidson, my editor—thank you for your steady eye, your care with language, and your commitment to keeping these pages both clear and compassionate. You helped shape this work with wisdom and grace.

To Hailee Pavey, for the art and cover design—thank you for giving visual beauty to such tender content. Your work captures the spirit of these pages in a way words alone cannot.

To Scott Guerin, my publisher—thank you for your support and your belief in the message behind this book.

To my beta readers, Paul Arrigo, Bella Dion, Bill Ehlig, Eleanor Perry Ford, Ivory JohnBaptiste, Catherine Larson, Rebecca Middleton, and Dwight Reagan—thank you for reading with honesty and heart. Your feedback helped refine these pages so they could better serve those who are grieving.

To those in the grief community who have shared their stories, questions, and quiet truths with me—thank you. You have taught me that grief is not something to "get over," but something we learn to live with, breathe with, and carry with love. Your courage helped shape these pages more than you know.

To my fellow God Talks Certified Coaches—thank you for your encouragement, your prayers, and the steady reminder that healing can be both spiritual and practical. Your support has meant more than I can put into words.

To David Kessler's Grief Educator Alumni Community—thank you for the wisdom, learning, and companionship you offer to those of us who serve grieving hearts. I am grateful for the depth, integrity, and care that lives within this community.

To the Lee College Grief Support Team—thank you for the sacred work you do and for being a steady presence for those walking through loss. I am grateful for your partnership, your compassion, and your willingness to make room for honest grief and real support.

To my family—thank you for your patience, your love, and the ways you have held space for me while I wrote words that were sometimes heavy to carry. Thank you for being part of the tenderness behind this book.

And to you, dear reader—thank you for trusting these pages. If you are holding this book in the midst of grief, please know that you are not alone. May these words meet you gently. May they steady your breathing. May they help you carry love forward, one quiet truth at a time.

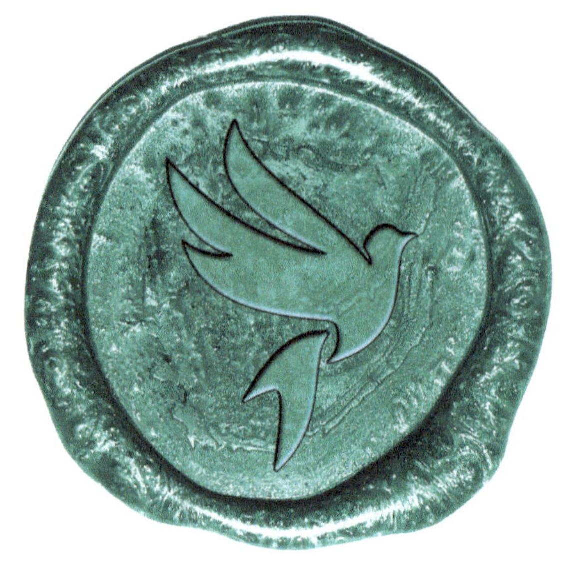

Help Is Always Available

Grief is a deep and personal process. It is very important that you have the support you need.

Grief can leave you feeling vulnerable and alone. Even kind people may say things that miss the mark. Professional support can help—but choose wisely. Look for a counselor trained in working with those in grief. Ask for referrals, interview prospective counselors, and trust your gut. It will recognize someone who feels safe, attentive, and respectful. Healing begins when you feel truly heard.

If you are feeling that life is not worth living or is more than you can handle, please contact a suicide or crisis hotline. Here are a few to choose from, available twenty-four hours a day:

- **Dial 988** to talk to a counselor at the 988 Suicide & Crisis Lifeline. All conversations are free and confidential.
- **Call 1-800-273-8255** to reach the National Suicide Prevention Lifeline.
- **Text HOME to 741741** to reach the Crisis Text Line.

Additional resources for your grief journey can be found at **LynetteRelyea.com.**

LYNETTE RELYEA

Transforming Grief into Strength, Wisdom, and the Quiet Wow

Certified Grief Educator

Access free downloadable resources from all of Lynette's books and explore her full range of products and services.

To discover more, visit

LynetteRelyea.com

Follow on Facebook:

LynetteRelyeaCertifiedGriefEducator

Connect on LinkedIn:

Linkedin.com/in/certifiedgriefeducator

Continue Supporting Your Grief Journey with The Wise Widow Collection

The Wise Widow Collection offers a tender and supportive path through grief. Whether read separately or side by side, these two books walk gently with you—honestly, compassionately, and at your own pace.

Conversations with the Wise Widow is a heartfelt companion for anyone navigating loss. Through personal stories and gentle reflections, it invites you to connect with your Wise Widow, breathe through the pain, and find your own way forward. This book offers comfort without clichés, strength without pressure, and the space to simply be with what you're feeling.

Your Wise Widow's Guidebook is a hands-on companion to *Conversations with the Wise Widow.* It provides thoughtful prompts, practical tools, and space to reflect, meeting you where you are. This guidebook offers gentle support and room to be honest as you move toward steadiness, grace, and peace on your healing journey. Your healing journey is your own—and this guidebook will help you walk it with intention.

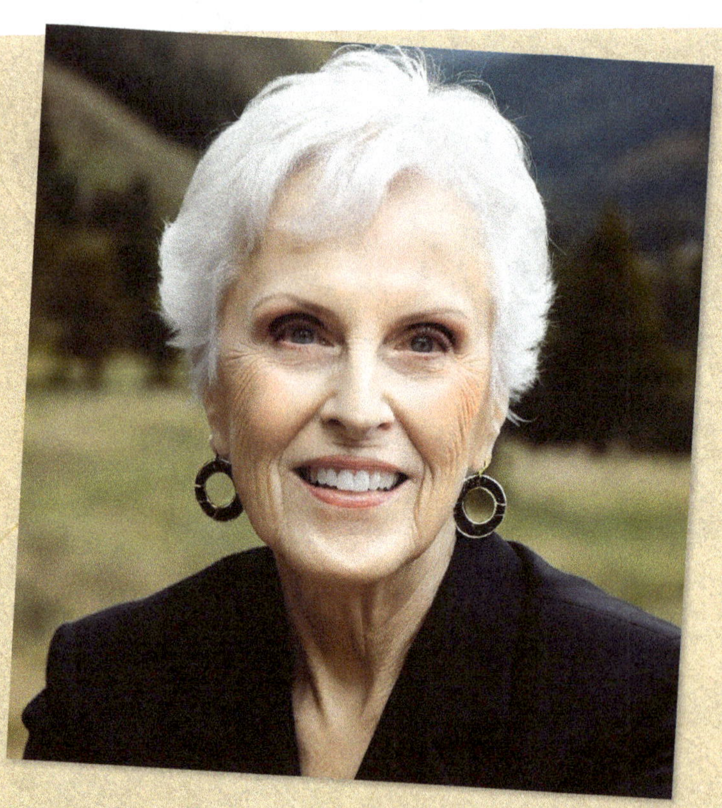

With love and presence,

Lynette Relyea

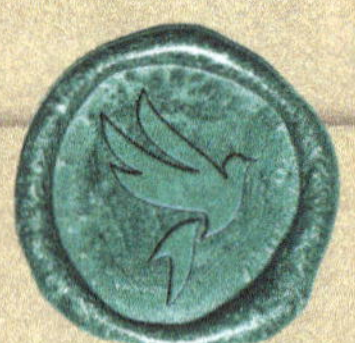

About the Author

Lynette Relyea is someone whose own grief ignited the belief that, after the loss of a Loved One, it is possible to do what feels impossible: keep living—without leaving love behind.

A certified grief educator, workshop facilitator, and creator of The Gift of Presence, Lynette is known for expressing complex grief experiences in language that feels steady, human, and deeply doable. Her work is rooted in a simple truth: grief doesn't need fixing—it needs presence. And when someone is met with calm, compassionate presence, the heart can begin to breathe again.

Lynette is the author of *Conversations with the Wise Widow: Transforming the Tsunami of Grief into the Quiet Wow* and *Your Wise Widow's Guidebook: Navigating through Grief to Healing, Strength, and Your Quiet Wow,* along with other grief-centered resources designed to support individuals, families, and communities.

With decades of experience as an educator in public schools and college classrooms, Lynette brings both clarity and compassion to grief support, offering practical frameworks that help people feel less alone, steadier, and more confident in life after loss.

Through her writing, workshops, and speaking, Lynette is building a movement that invites people to replace platitudes with presence, urgency with gentleness, and isolation with connection.

Healing doesn't mean forgetting. It means learning how to live forward—with love still intact.

www.ingramcontent.com/pod-product-compliance
Lightning Source LLC
LaVergne TN
LVHW010904110826
845149LV00005B/1461

* 9 7 9 8 9 9 9 0 3 9 1 5 6 *